MW00478548

DATE DUE

12-21-2 2	
1-1174-2023	

BEYOND THE
COTTONWOOD
TREES

For the community
of Cogir of Mill Creek.

Hunt
Bryce

BEYOND THE COTTONWOOD TREES

The Adventure Continues

HERB BRYCE with ANNA KATZ

HB BOOKS

Published by HB Books, Shoreline, WA
www.HerbBryce.com

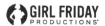

Edited and designed by Girl Friday Productions
www.girlfridayproductions.com

Cover design: Paul Barrett
Project management: Mari Kesselring and Reshma Kooner
Editorial production: Abi Pollokoff
All photos courtesy of the author, except: 19, Idea Lab;
119, TunnelTalk; 170, MOHAI (2000.107.171.17.01)

ISBN (hardcover): 978-1-7343885-6-5
ISBN (paperback): 978-1-7343885-4-1
ISBN (e-book): 978-1-7343885-5-8

Library of Congress Control Number: 2022909964

In loving memory of Gloria

TABLE OF CONTENTS

INTRODUCTION

On the Road to Adulthood

It's January of 1951. I'm seventeen years old, and I've just graduated from Compton High School, my tenth school since first grade. Besides a three-year stint at Avondale Elementary in Goodyear, Arizona, during World War II, when my dad worked at the Goodyear Aircraft Company, I moved pretty much every year—from my maternal grandparents' farm in Ashurst, Arizona, to wherever my parents' employment took us. Because I was always the new kid, and because my grandparents gave me both ample love and ample freedom, I had a strong independent streak and a very healthy dose of confidence.

What I didn't have was a clear-cut path forward. My grandparents, Nancy Lodema Mashburn Herbert and Lafayette Alexander Herbert, were farmers through and through; neither of them had finished elementary school. When my parents, Louise Herbert Bryce and Carlos Howard Bryce, went to Fort Thomas High School in the 1920s, they'd had two options for finishing secondary education. Option A was a four-year college prep curriculum, which culminated in graduation with a diploma. Option B was a three-year life-prep curriculum, which ended without a diploma. Girls took home-economics courses like cooking, sewing, millinery, laundering, home decoration, sanitation, and hygiene, while boys enrolled in wood and metal shop, auto mechanics, maintenance of machinery, and electrical and plumbing. Both of my parents chose option B.

Though my family didn't have much experience with formal higher education, they had always encouraged my curiosity. I was forever asking questions, reading books, and experimenting, taking apart and putting back together everything from car engines to milk separators. To them, my interests were practical—on the farm, you had to know how things worked so you could fix them when they broke. But ever since Mr. Kühn's fifth-grade science class, I'd known that I was going to be a scientist, not a farmer or mechanic (though the overlap between these vocations is significant).

Despite my benign troublemaking born of boredom and my bouncing from school to school, I'd excelled in class. After only one semester at Compton High School in Compton, California, the principal called me into his office. It was right before winter break, and the halls still echoed with the sound of lockers being gleefully slammed shut and the students calling out "Merry Christmas" to one another as they fled the building. It had been a while since I had mixed hydrogen and oxygen together in a balloon to create an extremely loud explosion or set off a smoke bomb—for the past few months, I'd managed to refrain from my usual pranks. Still, I couldn't help but assume that I was in trouble for something, even if I didn't know what.

To my surprise, the principal greeted me with a smile. Once I'd taken a seat, he reached across the desk and handed me a piece of paper. "Congratulations," he said. "Here's your diploma."

It took me a moment to collect myself. "Are you sure?" I asked. "What about the rest of the year?"

"Yes, I'm sure," he replied. He stood up. "Go to college," he said with a nod as we shook hands. "That's where you belong."

And so I would go to college. Of course, the route would not be straightforward. I would attend multiple schools and spend four years in the navy during the Korean War before earning a master's in natural sciences in 1962. There were no federal student loans, so I would do odd jobs to fund my education, working in roles from custodian to beekeeper, contractor to service station attendant to drugstore clerk.

My life was mine, I realized that moment in the principal's office, and I was responsible for it.

For those readers who are curious about the misadventures of my youth and growing up during some of the most pivotal times in America, from 1933 to 1951, I recommend my first book, *Me and the Cottonwood Tree*. That book ends where we now begin: in 1951, with the blank pages of my adulthood before me.

CHAPTER 1

A Big Fish in a Little Pond

And so, without ceremony, I'd graduated from high school. While my peers celebrated Christmas and the new year of 1951 with the comforting knowledge that they'd soon be returning to school and life would be carrying on as normal, I was looking ahead, toward the rest of my life, with excitement and confidence tinged with a touch of trepidation. *Adulthood, here I come!*

In the early spring, my football buddy Denzel Arrington from Mesa High School told me that he, Rae Brimhall, and LeRoy Ward had all gotten football scholarships at Arizona State College at Flagstaff (now Northern Arizona University). "If you had stayed at Mesa High instead of moving to Compton for senior year," he said, "I'm sure you could have gotten a scholarship, too. It would be great for the four of us to play together again."

Wow! A scholarship! Play the sport I loved and get a free ride to college to boot? How could I ask for anything more?

Right away, I reached out to the Mesa football coach, Coach Brady, who happened to have been a big star player at ASC-Flagstaff. He said he would be glad to write a letter of recommendation based on my performance during my junior year. I also contacted the head coach at Compton, who agreed to do the same for my senior year. I had two things going in my favor: we'd been the Arizona state champions my junior year at Mesa High, and during my senior year at Compton High, we had won the Southern California championship.

For some reason I cannot for the life of me recall, I asked my coaches to send their letters of recommendation to Brigham Young University instead of ASC. Perhaps I thought that a university was more prestigious than a college. Or it could have been that more than 99 percent of the student body at BYU belonged to the Church of Jesus Christ of Latter-day Saints, meaning I would avoid culture shock, and, more importantly, I would be automatically certified as safe to date. (Later someone pointed out to me that returned missionaries had the platinum certification and were the preferred catch.)

A few weeks later, I got a letter from the BYU coach offering me a tryout for a football scholarship.

Meanwhile, I was back in Mesa, working on my uncle Grant's bee farm, removing and melting down wax from old honeycomb frames and transporting hives to farms that had rented them. The pay was good, or at least good enough for me to put up with all the stings. With college football tryouts on the horizon, I gave Grant notice that my last day would be July 20 so that I could drive west to Compton, California, to spend a few days with my family before packing all my belongings into my army surplus footlocker, loading it into the trunk of my car, and heading out to BYU.

In 1951, there were basically two routes to Provo, Utah,

from Compton. One was through Las Vegas and St. George, then north on Route 91. The other was through Arizona via Route 66 to Flagstaff, then north just before Winona on Route 89 and across the Colorado River on the Navajo Bridge at Lees Ferry. The song "(Get Your Kicks on) Route 66" was spot on; I would soon get my kicks from a nice girl with big hazel eyes and a perfect amount of tomboy. Dang, Jenny was cute.

On the way to BYU, I stopped in Flagstaff, Arizona, for a visit with my three amigos Denzel, Rae, and LeRoy, who had just started the season at ASC-Flagstaff. The afternoon of my arrival, Denzel took me to football practice to meet Coach "Jiggs" Insley. Apparently, they had been feeding him a line about how great a player I was and said he needed me on the team, because the coach took one look at me and said, "Hell! The way the Mesa boys talk about you, I thought you would be wearing a red cape and have a big 'S' on your chest. What's wrong, couldn't find a phone booth?" I blinked, surprised by this greeting. He continued, "I'd like to see if you are as great as they say you are. Wanna try out for the team?"

"Oh, uh, um . . . I have an offer from BYU," I said. "Their tryouts begin next Tuesday."

"That's not a problem. Go to the locker room and tell Jim I sent you to get the gear to suit up. Then get back out and practice with the team. If you're half as good as the Mesa boys say you are, I might give you a counteroffer."

I must have been doing all right, because the coach had me play different positions so he could assess my strengths and weaknesses. At the end of the practice, as the rest of the team started a lap before heading to the locker room, he called me over.

"Take a lap and shower, Herb," he said. "Then stop by my office for a chat."

TEMPTATION

At this point, I still wasn't all that interested in playing for ASC. I was quite sure I could make the team at BYU—oh, the arrogance of a seventeen-year-old!—and that was good enough for me. That is, until I was crossing the road between the playing field and the locker room and heard a car horn. I turned my head to see a dark-blue 1941 four-door Plymouth with four girls in it parked on the side of the road. This, let me tell you, was a vision to behold.

One of the girls poked her head out of the back window and yelled, "Hey, Herb, I'm your date tonight. Come on over, let's get acquainted." As I walked toward the car, she got out and met me halfway. That's when I noticed her auburn hair; I've always been a sucker for redheads.

"Hi," she said, a smile lighting up her face. "I'm Jenny. Denzel told me that it's my responsibility to convince you to change your mind about BYU and stay here at Arizona State. He said that you and I are a perfect match because we're both self-made and independent."

Wow, I thought, *this should be interesting.* "I guess we'll see about that," I said. "I'm looking forward to getting to know you better, but I need to shower and talk with the coach first. I'll be back as soon as I can."

"I'll be here waiting," she replied before turning and walking away. To the other girls, I overheard her say, "What a hunk. Thank yoooouuu, Denzel!"

I wanted to yell back, *It's all football pads!* but I restrained myself, thinking, *Don't burst her bubble yet. She'll see me without my gear soon enough.*

After my shower, I got dressed, told the guys that I would be just a minute, and went to the office to talk with the coach. "Have a seat," he said, gesturing to one of the chairs in front of his standard-issue desk. He leaned back to sit on the desk's edge. "I'm impressed with your workout," he went on, casually folding his arms across his chest, "but I need some time to think about how you might fit in, and to talk to the other coaches. Promise that you won't leave for BYU before we talk again, OK?"

I nodded. I wasn't in a big hurry to rush off, now that I'd met Jenny. The coach looked past me over my shoulder at my buddies milling around in the locker room. "They waiting for you?" he asked. "Looks like they are getting impatient."

I turned in my seat; Denzel smiled and waved at us. "Yeah," I said. "There's a car full of girls parked outside. Denzel talked one of them into being my date tonight. She said her mission was to convince me to stay here."

"Good man. I'll see you tomorrow after lunch, at one o'clock. We'll talk over my offer. Now get out of here and have some fun. I hope she fulfills her mission."

I shook the coach's hand, then joined my buddies. Outside the locker room, the girls were waiting for us as promised. The car was designed for six people, with new blue-and-white vinyl bench seats front and back. Our party now totaled eight, with four of us big, broad-shouldered football linemen. "Why don't I go get my car?" I offered.

"No way," Jenny said. "I want to sit on your lap."

I shrugged, not too unhappy with this suggestion, and we all squeezed in.

"This is Carol," she said, nodding toward the driver, a tall gal with curly blond hair. "That's Betty in the middle, and this is Marilyn." She gestured toward the young lady sitting on LeRoy's lap by the passenger door. The two brunettes said hello.

"It's so hot out here," Marilyn said. "Let's go to the movies."

"Oh yeah!" piped in Betty. "I hear *Strangers on a Train* is good."

"I hear it's a nail-biter," Carol added. "You'll hold me tight if I get scared, won't you, Denzel?"

At the theater, we bought popcorn and headed for the balcony. We weren't the only ones who had thought to escape the July heat, and most of the seats were filled. It was a tense movie, and the audience was riveted, the only sound in the dark theater the munching of snacks and the slurping of soda.

Then, in a moment of silence, Jenny yelled out, "Hands off, Randolph! I'm only thirteen! Besides, the zipper is in the back."

The eight of us cracked up—until we heard someone running up the steps to our right. Jenny turned to me, grabbed my hand, and said, "It's the usher! Quick. Down the stairs to the left."

We pushed our way out and ran. Back in the lobby, we slowed down and caught our breath while trying to look nonchalant. *Nothing to see here, people.* Jenny looped her arm through mine and leaned in. "You just passed test number two," she whispered, her breath tickling my ear. "I'm getting to like you more and more."

"Me, too," I replied.

The next day at one o'clock, I returned to the coach's office to see what he had to say. "Well," he said, clapping his hands together, "we are prepared to offer you a full scholarship. That covers tuition, books and fees, room and board, and a job in the greenhouse. What do you say?"

That, plus my already established crew and the promise of a friendship with Jenny, made it impossible for me to refuse.

SLIDE DOWN TO THE END OF THE
BENCH FOR A BETTER VIEW

One thing that never entered my mind when I considered applying for a football scholarship was the college's enrollment size. I was aware that BYU had approximately 5,000 students. It was an utter surprise, however, when I found out that the enrollment at ASC-Flagstaff was 513. Yes, you read that right, it's not a typo: 513.

BYU's football roster boasted 57 players, compared to 29 for ASC-Flagstaff. Suddenly, I realized that, with such a meager student body and so few boys competing for a spot on the field, I had a chance to become a big fish in a very small pond.

That fall, our first game was at Highlands University in Las Vegas, New Mexico. A few minutes before game time, we gathered together in the locker room to listen to the coach read off the starting lineup. My stomach clenched in anticipation—I knew he had liked what he saw of my skill on the field, but would he put me in? When he got to my position, he paused, taking his eyes off the paper for just a moment to catch my eye.

"Right guard," he said, then called out last year's starting guard's name. I felt like I'd been socked in the gut. *They gave me everything but the kitchen sink just to sit on the bench?* I thought. Really what I should have been thinking was *You are the newest and youngest kid on the team, and Gene played that position last year. You are lucky as hell to even be here.*

The rules weren't what they are now, with a separate offense and defense platoon. All of us played both positions as needed. So, I sat on the bench feeling sorry for myself, watching the game, imagining that, if only Coach would let me play, I could get out there and kick some butt.

Finally, in the last half of the fourth quarter, I'd had enough. To Rae, I grumbled, "I should have gone to BYU instead of staying here."

The coach's head snapped up. Apparently, he'd heard me. With a grim look, he said, "You think you're better than Gene? Then get out there and prove it."

I nodded at Gene as we switched places, him removing

his helmet and swiping the back of his hand across his sweaty forehead. Here, now, was my chance.

I don't think I ever played so hard in my life.

After the game, the coach ran through his usual postmortem without mentioning me or my performance. But during practice on Monday, he kept moving me around to different positions, watching me, and taking notes. A week later, we headed over to New Mexico University for our next game. As we had the last time, we gathered together in the locker room to hear the starting lineup before the game. Again, when he got to my position, Coach paused. After an eternity, he said, "OK, Bryce, you think you can handle it?"

"Yes!" I shouted, then cleared my throat. In a calmer voice, I said, "Yes, I do."

"Then show me what you got."

Gene preferred to play tackle and was happy to switch so I could play running guard. I started every game for the rest of the season.

TWO TIMES FOUR

For the remainder of my time at ASC—which turned out to not be very long—the eight of us who went on that first trip to the movies became a tight group. Naturally, we coupled up, me with Jenny, Denzel with Carol, Rae with Betty, and LeRoy with Marilyn.

LeRoy and Marilyn made the oddest couple. He was nearly seven feet tall, and after football season, he played center on the basketball team, while Marilyn was the shortest of the bunch, coming up to his armpit when she stood on tiptoe. I suspected that they were together for sheer hilarity, running around campus like their own little comedy duo.

In the 1940s and '50s, colleges felt that it was their responsibility to protect the female students. There was a notable absence of a reception room in the men's dormitory, which seemed unnecessary given that women were not allowed to even step foot inside. We did, however, have fire escapes—perhaps the college administrators did not think that women could climb ladders.

The women's dormitory had two reception rooms with an attendant on duty to make sure no male gained entrance to the rooms beyond. They also enforced the curfews; the residents had better be home by ten p.m. Monday through Thursday, one a.m. Friday and Saturday, and midnight on Sunday, or else. Keep the girls locked up, was the thinking, and prevent hanky-panky. Instead of fire escapes with ladders, which a motivated male could climb, the women's dorm had fire poles outside a window at the end of the hall.

Do you have any idea how hard it is to climb a fire pole?

The city of Flagstaff was pretty dead as far as college students were concerned. The eight of us looked south to the Oak Creek Canyon area, thanks to Jenny, whose parents owned a cabin with an apple orchard across from what is now Sedona. I had some good memories of the area from when I was much younger, when I spent time there with my dad's sister Beulah and her husband, Colbert, who were taking care of two of Dad's brothers, Ed and Bill, and a sister, Flora, after their mother died. Ed was a year older than me. We played, swam in the creek, and skated in the Indian Gardens skating rink, which Beulah and Colbert owned.

Just getting there was an adventure. The two and a half miles of road descending and ascending the twelve-hundred-foot drop from the Coconino Forest plateau to the Oak Creek Canyon floor was treacherous. It was notoriously narrow, with one-foot shoulders and no safety railing or reflectors along the six switchbacks. My 1942 DeSoto's headlights were tungsten-sealed beams, ten times dimmer than those of today's cars. Of course, my young eyes were ten times better back then.

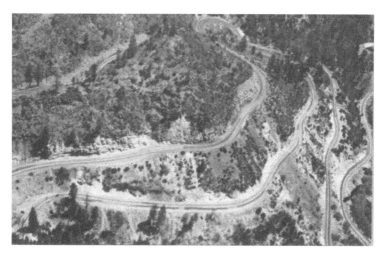

The famous switchbacks of Oak Creek Canyon

If that wasn't enough to tempt fate, the car had bench seats designed for three, not four, people in the front and three, not four, people in the back; no seat belts; a stick shift on the floor; and a Necker's knob on the steering wheel. To fit everyone, Denzel, Rae, and LeRoy would sit in the back seat, with Betty and Marilyn on their boyfriends' laps; in front, Carol sat by the passenger door and Jenny sat in the middle, her legs straddling the gearshift and my right arm around her shoulder, me driving with my left hand on the Necker's knob. I would tell Jenny the gear, and she would watch my left foot on the clutch pedal and change the gear for me.

We were teenagers and therefore invincible.

Back when I was a kid, the population of the area had been exceedingly small, with approximately one hundred residents. The population had recently swelled to more than ten thousand due to the discovery of a groundwater aquifer under West

Sedona in 1951. Natural artesian springs fed Oak Creek, which offered crystal-clear water to swim about in. Deep pools were perfect for cliff jumping, and a natural rock water slide next to the Pendley homestead offered hours of entertainment. (The State Parks Board acquired the Pendley homestead on July 9, 1985. Where we swam and played for free now has an entrance fee of thirty dollars per car for the day.) There were trails to explore and an outdoor firepit at the cabin to sit around talking and roasting wieners and marshmallows. We spent many an autumn night gathered around, laughing and carrying on until the wee hours of the morning.

Oak Creek was stocked year-round with rainbow trout, and it was also home to some beautiful carryover and wild rainbows. One Saturday, we decided to go fishing and cook dinner at Jenny's parents' cabin. As we were taking the fishing poles out of the trunk, I asked Rae if he wanted one. "No," he answered, "I'm going to lasso my fish."

I furrowed my brow in confusion. "What?" I said.

"I'm going to lasso my fish," he repeated.

"That's the craziest thing I ever heard."

Rae shrugged. "I've done it before." He smiled. "I'll show you how it's done."

"C'mon," I said, shaking my head. "I didn't just fall off the turnip truck."

"Oh yeah? I'll bet you a dollar that I can."

"I'll put money on that," LeRoy chimed in. The rest of the group added their dollars to the betting pool, too.

"Two conditions," Rae said, holding up two fingers. We looked at him, waiting expectantly. "One, no one can be in the water or casting shadows on the water upstream." We all nodded. "Two," he continued, "no loud noises." We all nodded again.

With that, Rae pulled a two-foot-long thin copper wire out of his pocket and bent it into a four-inch diameter lasso.

I looked over at Jenny, who rolled her eyes at me. "No way," she whispered. He then lay down on the bank at a curve in the river, where a scattering of rainbow trout was mulling about in the shallows. For a few minutes, he stayed motionless, holding the copper-wire lasso still in the water. We watched silently from a few feet back. Suddenly, he yanked his arm up, and, lo and behold, hanging in the loop, the wire tightly wrapped behind the thrashing fish's gills, was his dinner.

Never bet on a sure thing.

SURPRISE, GUESS WHO

In all my years playing football, my parents had never seen me play, not even when they lived within walking distance of the Compton High stadium.

So I was more than a little confused when, during the homecoming game at ASC, I made the tackle that every defensive player dreams of and heard a voice screaming, "That's the way to stop 'em, Brycey boy!"

Oh my God, I thought. *Is that . . . my mother?* I followed the direction of the voice and spotted her up in the stadium, where she was jumping up and down and waving her arms and yelling. Don't forget that, with a student body of 513, our stadium was smaller than a lot of high school stadiums. So it was easy to find someone hollering their head off and waving their arms like a lunatic.

Later I learned that Denzel had secretly called and persuaded them to come to the game. He bought them tickets and even had a homecoming mum waiting for Mom. I couldn't get my parents to walk five blocks to watch a game, but somehow Denzel had talked them into driving five-hundred-plus miles each way.

One thing Denzel hadn't factored in was that I had a date

with Jenny that night. I hadn't known I'd have visitors, so why wouldn't I? It was homecoming, after all. We had planned to get a bite to eat and then head to the dance. But Jenny was too well mannered not to take the opportunity to invite Mom and Dad to go to the café with us.

After the game, I took a quick shower and put on my freshly laundered Levi's and white button-up shirt, then raced outside. I didn't want to leave Jenny alone with my parents too long—who knew what kind of embarrassing stories my mom would be telling?

It was an interesting dinner. After my parents ordered chicken-fried steaks and my date and I ordered burgers and fries, Mom and Jenny tried to impress each other with their exceptional conversation skills, and Dad and I tried to get two words in edgewise. Terrified of the prospect of ending up at the dance as a foursome—my parents loved to dance, and my mom wasn't too shy to invite herself—I looked at Dad and pointedly raised my eyebrows; he finally caught the hint.

"Well," he said, standing and yawning theatrically, "it was a long drive from Needles this morning, and your mom and I should head to the motel to get some sleep."

"Oh really?" I said, trying to keep the glee from my voice.

Dad suppressed a smile, then continued, "Tomorrow morning, we're going to drive out to the Coconino Forest to see if we can find where we lived when you were just a kid."

"I didn't know you lived out there," Jenny said. "What part of the forest?"

"A few miles southeast of Mormon Lake."

"Well, it's been fun, but we have a dance to get to. Mom, can I help you with your coat?" I said, hoping to avoid what I knew was coming next.

"Do you want to go with us?" Mom said, dropping a bomb on my weekend.

"Sure," Jenny said, completely oblivious to the subtleties of this exchange. "Sounds like fun! And you can tell me all about what Herb was like growing up."

Believe me, Mom did and then some.

YOU'RE HERE FOR AN EDUCATION

For our Saturday games, the ASC football team traveled to schools in New Mexico, Idaho, and California; with only twenty-nine players, we only needed one bus. On Fridays, my English professor usually assigned essays to be turned in on Monday. Early on in that first semester, he pulled me aside to tell me that, when we played away games, I didn't have to turn in the essay on Monday.

That meant that I didn't need to write them, I concluded, making a self-serving logical leap. Boy, did I ever misunderstand him.

After the last game before Thanksgiving, the professor again pulled me aside. "Herb," he said, "finals week is coming up, and I've yet to see any of your essays."

Gulp.

"Right," I said, comprehension catching up with me like a punch to the gut. "I'm planning to get those to you this Monday."

I was truly thankful for Thanksgiving weekend. Thankful that the dorms emptied out and all my buddies went home. Thankful for Mother Nature's first snowstorm of the year covering Flagstaff with more than a foot of snow. Thankful for the snowplow stranding my car in a four-foot bank of snow. Thankful for the college's steam heating system that ran under the sidewalks, so I could get to the college's dining room. Thankful that there was nothing to distract me from writing.

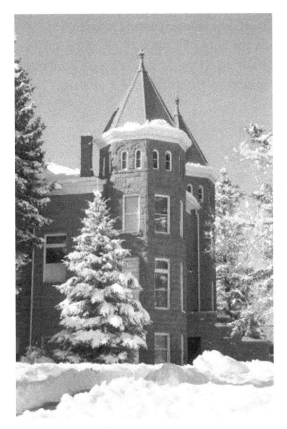

Snowy morning at Old Main

Nothing, that is, except for Jenny. She was one of the few students who lived in Flagstaff. When I told her about my predicament, she said that if I came for Thanksgiving dinner and stayed for the day, she would respect my writing time the rest of the weekend.

After a lovely dinner of roasted Brussels sprouts, home-made cranberry sauce, biscuits piping hot from the oven, and perfect golden-skinned turkey, Jenny went into her bedroom and came back with an eight-by-ten portrait of me.

"Will you sign this?" she asked, handing it to me.

I looked down at the photo. It was a photo of me, my hair parted neatly on the side and slicked into place with Brylcreem, my pensive gaze up and to the right. For a moment, I was

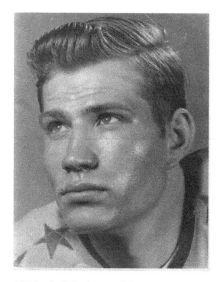

ASC football, freshman, 1951, age seventeen

confused. Where had she gotten it? Then I remembered that, before the first game of the season, Fronske Studio took portraits of each player on the team for the yearbook. "How'd you get this?" I asked.

Jenny grinned and gestured for me to carry on. I took the pen and, just as I was signing my name at the bottom of the photo, she said, "Well, wouldn't you know it, but Carol and Marilyn and I were walking down Aspin Avenue when who did we see on display at Fronske Studio? You, Denzel, LeRoy, and some of the other guys on the team. We went in and asked how much they cost, and they told us that we couldn't buy them without the permission of the player in the portrait. As we were leaving, we stopped for one more swoon. Then we were walking down the street and Carol tapped me on the shoulder and handed me the photo of you."

"Jen! Carol stole it!" I said. "Why didn't you take it back?"

Jenny cast her eyes down. "I wasn't the one who took it. And, anyway, I really wanted your picture! It's the last thing I see before I go to sleep and the first thing I see when I wake up in the morning."

The next day, I went to Fronske Studio and talked to the woman at the counter. "So a friend of mine took a photo of me . . . ," I began.

The woman took a good look at me. "Ah yes, I recognize you," she said. "When we noticed it was gone, we suspected that one of three college girls took it. When I'd told them that they had to get your permission, they weren't very happy."

"By the time I figured out she stole it, I'd already signed it, and it was too late to bring it back," I said, pulling my wallet out of my back pocket. "I'm sorry. I'm here to pay for it."

"The girl who took it should be the one apologizing and paying for it."

"Yeah, well . . . I want to pay for it."

I bought a birthday card, added "un" between "Happy" and "Birthday," and inserted the receipt. Then I gave it to Jenny.

DANCING ON A CLOUD

After that first snow of Thanksgiving weekend, the group moved our playground fifteen miles northwest, from Oak Creek to the San Francisco Peaks. The highest peak of the San Francisco Mountain range is 12,637 feet. While that might sound high, keep in mind that Flagstaff's elevation is 6,909 feet.

Arizona Snowbowl was established in 1938, making it one of the longest continually operating ski resorts in America.

None of us were skiers, so we played near the resort, making snowmen and snow angels and having snowball fights. We slid on flattened cardboard until we saw a couple of people flying down the hill on inner tubes.

When the Highway A89 switchbacks were cleared of snow, we would head to Jenny's parents' cabin. The Oak Creek area got very little snow, if any, no matter if it was storming in Flagstaff. We would bundle up and, just after the early winter sunset, we'd make a fire in the firepit and sip hot chocolate or hot apple cider and make s'mores.

The snow melted on the first of April. One chilly evening, the last of the day's light fading blue, Jenny and I and two other couples were in a favorite Flagstaff café. We'd finished our burgers and fries, and the other five had moved on to milkshakes for dessert. I was enjoying peach cobbler à la mode and a glass of milk.

"Hey," Carol said, dabbing at her chocolate milkshake mustache with a napkin. "Instead of skating at Indian Gardens in Oak Creek on Saturday, let's go to Cornville."

"Cornville? You gotta be kidding," said Denzel. He took a noisy slurp of his strawberry shake, then continued, "There's nothing in Cornville but a bunch of cattle ranches and a post office. They don't even grow *corn* in Cornville."

So why the name Cornville? Apparently, when the original settlers applied for a post office in 1887, they requested the name Cohnville in honor of a settler named Cohn. Washington sent the approval, but someone on the bureaucratic chain misspelled it, and the settlers, not wanting to take the trouble to reapply, accepted the mistake.

"No, really," Carol said, "there's a great dance hall over there. My uncle told me lots of stories about going to the dances when he was working at the copper smelter in Clarkdale. He'd tease my aunt, talking about all the pretty girls he danced with. He says the dance floor is built on car springs."

"What do you mean, car springs?" Jenny asked.

"Car springs, under the wood. He says it feels like dancing on a cloud. Let's go! There's a dance every Saturday with a live band, a good one."

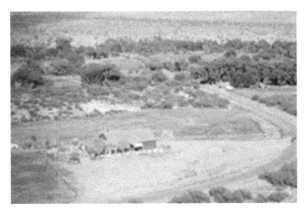

Cornville Dance Hall, 1952

"That sounds fun and all," I said, "but it's a bar and we're all under twenty-one. They're not going to let us in."

"It won't be a problem. My uncle started working at the smelter right after high school and got married when he was twenty. He was going there before he was married. Anyway, they serve only beer, no booze, so they're not so strict."

Turned out the music was great, as promised, and the car-spring dance floor did feel like dancing on clouds.

Many, many years later, I looked up the Cornville Dance Hall on this magical invention called the internet. Though I could not find the date it was built, the floor design and the bootlegging in the parking lot—where you could get that booze they wouldn't serve inside, if you were so inclined— led me to assume that it had been built in the 1920s, during Prohibition. A man by the name of Harley Thompson recalled how he and his dad would drive their Model A up into the Mingus Foothills, where known bootlegger John Zemp had a still and made "good bootleg whiskey." They would get a five-gallon tin, and, at home, they would take it down into the cellar and use a funnel to fill pints and half-pints that could fit inside coat pockets. They would sell these in the parking lot. Sadly, the Cornville Dance Hall burned to the ground on October 27, 1971.

Twenty years before that, Cornville Dance Hall became our go-to for Saturday nights. Jenny was a fantastic dancer. During Joe Garland's "In the Mood" or Vaughn Horton's "Choo Choo Ch'boogie," I would swing her over my back and then slide her along the floor between my legs. The slow dances were written just for us. With her head resting on my chest, I held her close to Walter Gross and Jack Lawrence's "Tenderly" or George and Ira Gershwin's "Embraceable You."

The dance hall was notorious for fighting—with so little else going on in the area, I guess people saw it as a place to be used efficiently for both hooking up and duking it out, fueled by beer or bootleg booze. A deputy sheriff stood by the entrance and would stop any fight that broke out inside or near the front door, only to usher the dispute out to the parking lot to finish. The fights were not limited to men.

Our little group stayed inside during intermission and went home early to avoid the chaos. We were lovers, not fighters.

UNCLE SAM WANTS YOU

A couple of weeks before I turned eighteen and a half, in late April 1952, I got a letter from the president. Back in my room, I ever so gingerly laid a damp washcloth on the sealed flap of the envelope.

The United States had been at war—sometimes euphemistically called "military conflict"—with North Korea for two years, since 1950. On June 25 of that year, the Korean People's Army crossed the 38th parallel, thereby breaching the line of peace between Soviet-occupied Korea to the north and American-occupied Korea to the south. The United States, afraid of a Communist takeover, jumped in to not only reinstate the boundary but to "free" the North Koreans.

The draft began right away, and would, over the course of the three-year conflict, induct more than 1.5 million people. In parts of Arizona, some draft boards and the LDS Church were competing in a game of first dibs. If you were called on a mission before you got drafted, you would be classified as 4-D, minister of religion, and exempt from service. Since I had decided not to attend BYU and had no plans to go on a mission, there was no chance I was going to get that classification.

Most draftees were conscripted into the army; the rest went into the marines. I, for one, could not imagine shooting at some guy my age who was supposed to be my enemy but probably wanted the exact same things out of life that I did. I remembered, as a kid, watching a movie about World War II and how the Germans were praying for victory. "So," I asked one of my uncles, "if the Germans are praying, and we're praying, then who is God listening to?"

"God is listening to us," he replied.

"Why?"

"Because we're right."

Just as my mother's explanation for why we were sending Japanese Americans to internment camps but not German Americans—namely, that German Americans looked like us—didn't make sense to me, my uncle's answer left a lot to be desired. Only a few years later, I still didn't understand. I had never heard the word "pacifist," though I suppose that was what I was. So I had one option: those of us who did not want to sleep in foxholes, eat K rations, and dodge bullets were enlisting in the navy. That is, if we could find a recruiting office that had openings.

After a while, the flap loosened, and I was able to nudge open the envelope without tearing it. Just as I feared, it was an order to report for induction.

I made sure that everything was replaced properly in the envelope and resealed it. When my roommate returned from class, I asked him to write *Enlisted in the Navy* on the front and post it a week after I dropped out of college and said my goodbyes.

The first naval recruiting center I stopped at was in Arizona, and I was informed that they didn't have an opening and were not taking any new recruits. Even if they did have an opening, they couldn't enlist me because I was sent a draft notice. But just as I was about to turn away and make my exit, the recruiting officer motioned for me to lean in. "If I were you," he whispered, "I'd head for California."

I followed his advice. At the fourth recruiting center in California, I finally was able to sign up. Jenny cried when I told her the news.

CHAPTER 2

Anchors Aweigh

Coach tried to convince me not to leave. It wasn't that he wasn't patriotic; rather, he just didn't want to lose any players. And there's nothing more American than football, right?

Denzel, Rae, and LeRoy agreed. Denzel put water in one ear and plugged it up for a couple days in order to make it inflamed before his physical exam. Rae put P&G laundry soap under his arm and left it there for three days, a trick to induce high blood pressure. LeRoy told the recruiter that he had blown out his knee, a complaint that, coming from an athlete over seven feet tall, was none too hard to believe.

But I didn't feel right about fibbing, even though I wasn't gung-ho about the war. I'd received two guns for Christmas when I was nine years old, and I'd never quite recovered from my guilt over killing a bird for no other reason than I could. So the navy it had to be.

At the third recruiting office I visited, the recruiter yet again told me that they were not taking recruits. He paused, squinting at me as though in thought. "You're in college, aren't you?" he said.

"Yes," I replied.

"Your major?"

"Physical sciences."

"Hold on a minute." I stood there as the recruiter dialed the rotary phone. "Jim?" he said into the handset. "I got a college boy here looking for a spot." I swallowed, getting my hopes up. The recruiter nodded a couple times, saying "uh-huh" and gazing out the window at the bland California day. Then, he said, "He wants to talk to you." He handed me the phone.

"Hello?" I said. "Herb Bryce speaking."

"Son," said a gravelly voice, "what's your educational background?"

"I've finished one year of college. My major is physical sciences."

There was a brief pause on the line. I held my breath.

"I've got one opening. It's in Naval Air, and you will need to pass a test. Interested?"

"Yes, sir."

"Come on down to the Downey recruiting office. You got two hours? You'll need to take a test."

"Yes, sir."

I hustled over to Downey. Was I nervous? Well, I was good at tests, but a little bit more than a grade was at stake here. I tried to put the prospect of getting shipped off and shot at out of my mind as I sat down in the little corner office with my sharp No. 2 pencil. The recruiting officer sat behind his desk just outside the door.

One hour and forty-five minutes later, I got up with a sigh and handed him the test. He nodded and pulled out the dreaded red pen. "You may go back into the office and sit down," he said. "I'll be with you shortly."

I did as told. There was no window to look out of, so I sat

back, twirling the pencil between my fingers. After a quarter of an hour, the recruiting officer stepped into the doorway.

"You did great," he said. "Only missed one question." I didn't realize that I had been holding my breath until I took a big inhale with the news. "Before you sign up," he continued, "you need to know what you are signing up for." He went over the standard information, reciting it in a way that let me know he'd given the same spiel many times before, then went into the specifics. "This position is for Naval Air only—no submarines or ships, though you could be on an aircraft carrier. It's more likely you will be on air bases, in the US or overseas."

I nodded, relieved that he hadn't mentioned Korea.

"Oh, and one other thing."

I looked up, afraid my luck had run out.

"With a year of college and your test score, you can enter as an E-3, an airman."

No anchors aweigh for me. All the bases at which I would be stationed were either a Naval Air school or a Naval Air base on dry land (except when it rained). The only exception was during the seventh week of boot camp, when we had classes on a two-thirds-scale mock-up of a destroyer escort parked on California soil. In 1949, this "non-ship" ship had been commissioned USS *Recruit* (TDE-1) to be used to teach traditional naval shipboard procedures, operations, and shipboard lingo.

I was inducted in Los Angeles on May 6, 1952, at eight a.m. It only took two days to go from being a civilian to being a sailor. After our physical exam, which involved stripping down, going from station to station for various assessments, answering questions about our sexual orientation, and peeing in a tube, we boarded a bus that took us to the Naval Training Center San Diego. There we lined up in rows and met our division commander, who gave us marching orders to the chow hall for a lunch of chicken, steamed broccoli, baked potato, and green salad, all piled high on stainless-steel trays, plus a big spoonful of chocolate pudding for dessert. We spent the afternoon taking several exams. "Do your best," the division commander told us, "because the better your scores are, the better your job will be." No pressure.

After a few grueling hours of exams, we were marched off to our new home, a big, open barracks with forty-eight bunk beds, each with a four-inch mattress folded in half and topped by two white wool blankets, a mattress cover, a small pillow and two pillow covers, and a ditty bag with the minimum necessities—a sewing kit, toiletries, personal items such as writing paper and pens, and a carton of Lucky Strike cigarettes. "I don't smoke," I told the division commander, holding out the box.

"Keep them," he said. "Lock them up in your seabag." Seeing the incredulous look on my face, he added, "Believe me. About a week before you go on liberty, the heavy smokers will be offering you ten dollars a pack."

The market rate for a pack was about a quarter, and I couldn't believe anyone would pay such a ridiculous price. Still, I wasn't totally opposed to a little profiteering, and immediately I sold mine off for five dollars each.

Reveille was at 05:00 the next day. We were given one hour to take care of our morning hygiene, to shave, shower, and dress, and properly make the bed, and be in formation and standing at parade rest. At 06:00, we heard "atteenHUT, forward—MAAARCH," and we were herded to the mess hall. After a breakfast of scrambled eggs, British baked beans, hot biscuits with butter and jam, and bacon and sausage, we were marched off to uniform supplies and issued our uniforms, seabag, and a bag with a drawstring and name tag. We stenciled our names and service number on our bedding and ditty bag, and marked our new shoes and socks with our initials. Every stitch of clothing, including our skivvies, had to have our identification on it in a specific location so that when rolled and tied in a particular way, the name and service number would show. Our last name was on our shirts' right front pocket and the back pocket of our dungarees. If we were found wearing anything without a stencil, we were told we would get court-martialed. The bag with the drawstring was for our civilian clothes, jewelry, pocketknife, and other unapproved items, and on its tag, we wrote our home addresses so the navy could mail it home. Dropping the bag of civilian clothes into the canvas bulk basket hit me hard—now I belonged to the navy.

To really seal the deal, we were then marched over to the barbershop. Inside were ten chairs with ten barbers standing behind them, electric shavers at the ready. I sat down in the first available seat. There was no mirror, so I couldn't take one last look at my spiffy blond hairdo.

In the middle of the room stood a stool with a white hat on it. "What's that?" I asked my barber. "You'll see," he said. Once all ten seats were filled with nervous-looking recruits, the barbers walked over and threw fifty-cent pieces into the hat. Then one of them said, "Ready . . . set . . . go!"

Well, turns out that whoever cut hair the fastest won the pot. You can imagine what that haircut looked like.

Unlike the other services that had footlockers in boot camp, we lived out of a twelve-by-thirty-six-inch heavy canvas seabag with a steel cable and padlock. Once a week, we had "seabag inspection," meaning that we had to lay out the contents on our bed in a specific manner. All clothing had to be tightly rolled and tied with clothes "stops," an eighteen-inch-long cord with brass tips, with our stenciled names and service number showing.

Back then, there were no ifs, ands, or buts about vaccination—meaning we couldn't opt out, as some of the military did for the coronavirus vaccine. We were given ten different vaccinations while in boot camp: cholera, influenza, plague, smallpox, tetanus-diphtheria, typhoid, typhus, paratyphoid A and B, and yellow fever. (As a matter of fact, I got a second round of shots when I was transferred to Litchfield Park Naval Air Facility in Arizona in 1953. I got a notice to report to sick bay; my vaccination records had been lost when I transferred from Millington, Tennessee, and I needed to restart my vaccination program.)

There were ninety-six recruits in our division. Because I was an E-3 and the rest of the recruits were E-1s, I was appointed recruit chief petty officer, the primary recruit assistant to the recruit division commander. In plain English, as RCPO I was in charge when the RDC went home. For that additional responsibility, I earned more money than the E-1s, at fifty-two cents per day. Whoopie! But being a glorified "manny" was not worth the fifty-two cents. My primary duties included: talking down recruits who were having buyer's remorse over their new tattoos, stopping skirmishes, quieting drunks, getting someone to sick bay in the middle of the night. Consoling recipients of "Dear John" letters was a big one—I was amazed at the number of these breakup letters. At least a third of my fellow seamen received one, and those are just the ones I heard about.

On Sunday mornings, all ninety-six companies—well over a thousand sailors—marched out to the parade field and lined up. The battalion officer from the chaplain's office would say over the loudspeaker, "All Catholics, take one step forward!" and, once all Catholics had, he'd holler, "Right face, forward march," and off they'd march to the Catholic church. Then it was the Protestants' turn. There was no Mormon church on base, and Jews were excused from duty to attend Shabbat services on Saturdays, so the other outliers and I were instructed to return to our barracks and read our Bibles. Over the next few weeks, recruits started losing their religion so that they, too, could spend the morning away from the watchful eyes of the navy and the church.

Boot camp in San Diego was fourteen weeks long. We

spent three weeks at the naval training center, three more weeks at Camp Elliott, then back to the NTC for the last eight weeks. We were quarantined on base until the last six weeks, during which we had one liberty day per week, alternating Saturday and Sunday.

If I'd exercised a little patience and waited to sell my cigarettes, I could have doubled my money, just as the division commander had predicted.

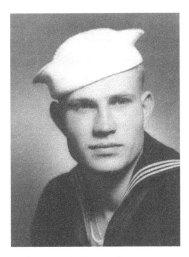

Herb Bryce, 1952, age eighteen

SURPRISE VISIT

After graduating from boot camp, we were granted leave for up to one month, depending on where we were headed next. I was the only one in Naval Air in our division, and I had to cut my leave short to be transferred to Norman, Oklahoma, to attend an Aviation Navy Preparatory (ANP) school.

Thirty-three men and I boarded a bus that took us to San Diego's Lindbergh Field to catch the DC-3 twin-prop airplane the navy had chartered. As we were getting off the bus, the pilot came over to talk with the chief petty officer who was escorting us. All of us strained to listen. "We've had some mechanical problems with one of the engines," he said. "We need to make repairs before we can leave."

It seemed like years before we were finally granted liftoff into the robin's-egg blue of the San Diego sky. Everything was A-OK as we flew northeast, leaving behind the salty breezes of the coast and heading over the desert toward the plains of Oklahoma. Though I'd had a couple weeks off, I was still tuckered out from boot camp, and the roar of the engines soon lulled me to sleep.

I woke up when my stomach crashed into my throat. I looked around the cabin, confused. My ears were plugged. The plane seemed to be tilted at an odd angle. I shook my head to try to clear it.

Oh my God, I thought, realization dawning. *We're diving.*

I couldn't hear a motor. I looked out my window and saw that the propeller was not rotating. My heart seized with panic. *I'm too young to die,* I thought. *Think of all the girls I haven't kissed!* Just as I had that regret, my ears popped, and I heard the engine on the other side, the propeller buzzing. No words can explain the relief I felt.

The plane landed safely at Childress, Texas, at 3:18 a.m. according to the local newspaper. Childress was a small town, with a population of seven thousand. The nearest naval base is Corpus Christi, Texas, more than five hundred miles away, so sailors in uniform were an unusual sight. Imagine waking up to find thirty-four bleary-eyed young sailors in dress blues wandering the streets looking for breakfast.

After a meal at one of the town's few cafés, some of us found the high school. The high school boys seemed interested at first, but they quickly decided that the girls were maybe a little too interested in these sailors who had magically appeared overnight. Meanwhile, we thought we had discovered paradise.

Childress High School was the only high school in the county; it had an enrollment of about three hundred students. You do the math: there were only seventy-five junior and senior girls in the whole county, which is not enough for both a group of sailors and the local teenage farm boys. I had noticed that most of the pickups in the school's parking lot had rifles hanging in a rack in the back window, and so when the insulting, pushing, and shoving began, and when the high school boys began pulling their girlfriends away by the arm, I realized it was time to go back into town.

Besides that hormone-fueled tension, the people in Childress were incredibly open and seemed to truly appreciate our serving our country. As I walked the block that made up the downtown, many approached to start a conversation. "What are y'all doing here?" more than one person asked. I gave them the basic rundown, minus the details of what I had considered to be our near-death experience, and told them we were headed to a navy base in Norman, Oklahoma. "There's a navy base in Norman?" they asked, incredulous. "As far as I can tell, that's a long way from the ocean."

Within the hour, I'd secured myself an invitation to a family dinner. A couple of elementary-school-age boys greeted me at the door, excited to see a real live sailor. I didn't miss the fact that the delicious dinner of deep-fried chicken, mashed potatoes and gravy, baked beans with ham hock, and salad was served by the lady of the house and her teenage daughter. Over dessert of chocolate-chip cookies and milk, I asked if the girl's boyfriend was one of the boys in the group at the high school.

"No," she answered shyly, her gaze averted. "I don't have a boyfriend. I just turned sixteen, though"—she snuck a glance at me—"so now I can start dating."

"She's not going to date until she's eighteen," her father said, a humorous and teasing smile playing on his lips.

After dinner, they took me back to town. The aircraft

charter company had arranged for an aviation mechanic and parts from Dallas to come to fix the engine, but in the meantime, someone had figured that it was cheaper to lease a bus than house and feed thirty-four sailors plus the two petty officer escorts. I'm sure the boys of Childress were more than happy to see our taillights as we drove off into the night.

PLEN'Y OF HEART . . .

My company was the first class at the ANP school when it reopened in 1952, after a five-year hiatus, in order to provide the technical training needed for the latest war. Our barracks was one of the original buildings built in 1942 to expand the Naval Air training capacity during World War II. (It closed for good in 1959.) The base was adjacent to the University of Oklahoma, its front gate opening onto a road that ran behind a women's dormitory.

Because of the age and wood composition of the building, we had fireguards overnight, from taps to reveille, made up of four non-officer groups of watch duty. There were no smoke alarms—we were the smoke alarms. We would have a twenty-four-hour stint on duty restricted to the base, then three days with liberty, which meant we could travel within a certain radius and, if desired, request special permission to go outside that radius. The commanding officer had the authority to set and change the times and rules concerning liberty, but usually workday liberty was from 16:00 to 07:59, and weekend liberty was from Friday 16:00 to 07:59 Monday morning. We had liberty cards that were color coded for the four groups.

On my first non-liberty day, I was assigned to be a fireguard. That night, with the only sounds in the barracks the heavy breathing and occasional snore of thirty-three sleeping men, I sat alone, ready to sound the alarm if need be. To stay awake, I decided to do some long-neglected correspondence. I'd been avoiding contacting Jenny—remembering her tears when I so abruptly said goodbye gave me a funny feeling in my heart. Now, with hours of quiet ahead of me, I knew that it was time to reach out.

I took the pen and paper out of my ditty bag and spread a fresh sheet out on the table in front of me. *Dear Jenny,* I wrote, then stopped. The last time I'd seen her, four and a half months earlier, I had held her hand while telling her I was leaving. "I understand," she'd said, looking up at me with those big hazel eyes, a watchful expression on her face. She'd turned away and swiped underneath her eyes with her thumbs, her breath catching. I'd given her hand a squeeze and then let it go; now I realized that she had been waiting for me to say . . . something. Anything. Maybe she was hoping for some kind of promise, or maybe she just wanted to hear a kind word, to know that she had meant something to me. Whatever it was, I had failed to deliver.

The lamp cast a yellow light on the mostly blank page. Now that I had the time and space to take an inventory of myself, I didn't like what I was finding. *I'm sorry for not writing sooner,* I began. I paused again. This was a lot harder than I thought it would be. I should have written her when I was in boot camp or during my brief leave. I put the pen down, cracked my knuckles, took a deep breath, picked the pen back up, and let the words flow.

The more I wrote, the more I realized what a jerk I was. Jenny had been my best friend, and I had hurt her. She wasn't the only one. The more I wrote, the more I realized what a jerk I'd been so many times, how I just walked away from friends whenever I moved. The longest I had ever lived in the same place was three years, and I had gotten so used to leaving people behind that I behaved thoughtlessly, even hard-heartedly, to protect myself. I'd developed a callus on my heart after losing friends over and over—it was painful to get close to people only to leave, and it was so difficult to maintain that closeness as I went from place to place. But that was no excuse.

By the time I finished the letter, it was more than an hour past the time for my relief to start. I didn't wake him; I worked his shift for him. It gave me more time to think about my behavior and what I needed to do to change.

I sent Jenny the letter but never heard back. I don't know if it was because she was angry with me or if she was heartbroken or if she'd moved on or if she simply didn't receive it. In the spring of 1953, when I was stationed in Arizona, I asked Denzel about Jenny.

"Does she . . . ever talk about me?"

He shrugged. "Every time your name comes up, she either changes the subject or walks away."

"Oh," I said, disappointed.

"Anyway, last I heard, she's engaged."

OH, WHAT A BEAUTIFUL MORNING

The function of the ANP school was to let us try out the duties of the different "rates," the navy's term for jobs. More importantly, it gave the navy an indication of where we would best fulfill its needs. At the end of term, I meet with the chief petty officer, who said, "We feel that the best rate for both you and the navy is one of the following three: tradevman, tradevman, or tradevman. Which do you think is best for you?"

"Huh," I replied. "Let me think this over . . . I'll take the second one, sir."

In case you are wondering whether that "v" is a typo, it's not. Tradevman (TD) stands for "training devices man." Yes, the name is sexist, though it was an ideal rate for women as well as men. The rate was established in 1948, and a very small number of us took on that role. Our job was to install, operate, maintain, and repair training devices. (When I was discharged in 1956, I was replaced with a civilian. They felt that hiring civilians was cheaper because they didn't have to provide all the perks given to military personnel. The rate was discontinued in 1988.)

The musical *Oklahoma!* got it right. "Plen'y of heart" well described the people I encountered while I was stationed in Norman. The U of OK football team was number four in the nation, so extra tickets could have sold at a top price, yet folks gave me and other sailors free tickets to every home game. As a recently retired football player, I took it upon myself to coach from the stands, but I guess the linemen and linebackers didn't hear me. Hitchhiking to Oklahoma City was easy, and often the waitress would slide me a slice of apple pie or chocolate cake, on the house, at whatever café I patronized for lunch. On a number of occasions, I was offered a home-cooked dinner and a ride back to the base by my fellow football fans.

Best of all was my friendship with Barbara.

It was my first free Saturday, and I woke up whistling, looking forward to liberty for the entire weekend. I ate the free breakfast at the chow hall, then headed out for my self-guided tour of campus. I found the chemistry building at the edge of Parrington Oval, a beautiful expanse of lawn dotted by trees. The president of the university had earned a reputation for his enthusiastic tree planting, and he'd silenced any complaints when he revealed that he'd paid for them out of his own pocket. Anyway, they were beautiful. I took a seat on a bench, content to look at the red and yellow autumn foliage and watch people. The students were friendly, some saying "good morning" and some just saying "hi" or waving as they passed. A few stopped to chat for a couple of minutes.

Then Barbara walked into my life. One look—her short curly ginger hair, brown eyes, fresh face with a light sprinkling of freckles across the bridge of her nose, and a bare ring finger on her left hand—caught my full attention. "Hi!" I said, all smiles. "Are you a student here?"

"Yes," she replied, her eyes sparkling. "Are you stationed at the base?" Her smile was wide and genuine; I knew I was a goner. I slid over to make more room on the bench and tapped the spot next to me. She took the hint and sat down facing me with her legs crossed.

We talked for more than an hour. She was an anthropology major, not just pretty but sharp as a tack. "Will you be my tour guide?" I asked as morning turned toward noon.

"I'd like that."

I stood up and offered my hand to help her up. Once she was standing, I didn't want to let go, so we walked hand in hand as she pointed out buildings and provided commentary.

"That building over there is the DeBarr chemistry hall," she said. "That's where you will be spending most of your time when you get out of the navy."

"Oh yeah? What makes you think I would want to come back?"

"Because I'll be here." She smiled.

"You're a sophomore, though. By the time I get out, you'll be in grad school."

"I'll still be here."

A few minutes later, we passed another grand building. "Other than my dorm, I spend most of my time here, for my anthropology classes."

"When are you going to show me your dorm?"

"When you bring me home tonight."

"How about lunch first?" We left campus, still holding hands, and strolled along the few short blocks to downtown. The air was warm but with a breeze, and a soft autumn light had replaced the harsher light of summer. After a couple of sandwiches and some iced tea, we toured the city, ending up in a nearby park. I sat down on the grass underneath a dogwood tree and leaned back, putting my weight on my elbows. Barbara lay down perpendicular to me and rested her head in my lap. We talked all afternoon as clouds floated across the clear blue sky. Occasionally one of us would stop midsentence to point at a cloud in the shape of a dog or a snowman or a duck.

At dinner, I finally worked up the nerve to ask her a question that had been on my mind all day. "Do you have a boyfriend?" I asked.

"Well," she said, dabbing the corners of her mouth with her napkin, "my high school boyfriend got a scholarship to Cornell. Engineering. As the adage goes, absence makes the heart grow fonder."

"I see."

She lay her napkin across her lap and smiled. "In this case, his heart grew fonder of someone else. Last spring break, he went to Florida to relax on a beach with his new girlfriend instead of coming home."

"Oh." I did my best not to grin. "If you don't mind my saying so, he sounds like an idiot."

Dusk was falling by the time we got to her dorm, her hand starting to feel familiar in mine. "I had a wonderful time," I said. "Thanks for spending the day with me."

Barbara turned to face me. "Can I take you to breakfast tomorrow?" she asked. "I can't remember enjoying just being with someone like I did today. I've got more questions I want to ask you."

"Want to ask me now?"

"No. I'd rather keep you wondering. And it's more fun laying my head in your lap. Pick me up at nine?"

Without thinking, I eagerly accepted. The short walk back to the barracks gave me time to ponder. I'd thought Barbara was attractive the moment I saw her, and she only got more so as the day went on. She was easy to talk with, to laugh with, to tease and be teased by. We enjoyed being together. She was witty, bright, and fun. What more could I ask for?

Reality hit when I got to my bed. My whole life could fit in a couple bags, bags that would feel light thrown over my shoulder when the time came to head out. *I'm going to be transferred in seven weeks to another base,* I thought, *and God only knows where and for how long.* Barbara had just been dumped by her boyfriend, and I did not want to risk hurting her so soon after that. Thoughts of Jenny and how I screwed up that relationship flooded my mind. *I cannot do that to Barbara. I cannot do this.*

There were no cell phones in 1952. All thirty-four of us plus the petty officer in charge shared one phone, guaranteeing zero privacy and likely at least one or two guys waiting in line. Anyway, I hadn't asked for her phone number, since we'd already made a date.

The next morning, I met her at her dorm at nine o'clock sharp. Over a breakfast of eggs and toast, I brought up the issue of my leaving. "I really like you," I told her, determined to let her know how I felt even though, in the end, my feelings wouldn't lead to promises. "But I'm leaving in a few weeks."

"You think we should just be friends, right?"

I nodded. "Yeah, I think so."

Barbara took a bite of toast and chewed thoughtfully. "Does that mean you don't want to see me again?" she finally said.

"I do want to see you again. Do you think we can keep it just friends?"

"Might as well try."

For the next seven weeks, we held hands as we wandered the tiny town of Norman, and every time I left her in front of her dorm, I gave her a warm hug good night. We were able to just be friends, but we were crazy to think we could stop our feelings for each other from growing stronger.

As the days got colder and the nights got longer, I left for

Millington, Tennessee, to attend tradevman school for twenty-two weeks. It was hard to say goodbye to Barbara. The good-bye kiss made it even more difficult. We exchanged letters for about three months, the time between each letter getting longer until, finally, she did not reply.

CHAPTER 3

Memphis, Here I Come

Barbara and I said our goodbyes while the bus driver loaded my
seabag into the luggage bay. He boarded and, after a moment,
tooted the horn. I kissed Barbara for the last time and tried
to memorize her face as I gave her hand a squeeze. My heart-
strings were tugging at me, telling me to stay. My mind was
telling me that I had to go, that I belonged to Uncle Sam now.

I found a window seat on the right-hand side of the bus so
I could get one last look at Barbara. She waved as we pulled out
of the station, her smile belying the sadness in her eyes.

From Norman, the bus headed north to Route 66 at
Oklahoma City. I was asleep by the time we reached Amarillo,
Texas, and I slept like the dead as we drove west through the
night, waking early in the morning when the bus went over
a particularly big bump. I was happy to disembark late that
afternoon in Los Angeles, my back stiff and my heart sore. I
got to my folks' place just in time for dinner. My mom made
my favorite treat—two of her famous lemon-cream meringue

pies, one for me and the other for her, Dad, and my two sisters to share.

My dad and I fished almost every day while I was home. He was a devout angler, and on one afternoon, he caught twenty-two halibut and one yellowtail compared to my single halibut. We were one of the few families with a freezer, and Dad put the haul away while Mom cooked up enough fish for dinner, plus another couple of her delicious pies. After months of navy chow, I was happy to get some home-cooked meals.

Eight days later, I boarded a train to Memphis. In Amarillo, Texas, the train stopped and hooked onto a milk car. Back then, milk trains would stop at dairy farms and pick up ten-gallon cans of milk and haul them to a dairy processing plant. Each full can weighed eighty-eight pounds and was manhandled—in other words, no machinery was used. When the train reached the processing plant, the train switched to a side track and the milk car was left there. That speeded things up.

When we got to Tulsa, Oklahoma, the car I was in was switched over to another train that was headed to Memphis. Twenty minutes after departure, I saw a light flashing through the windows and looked outside to see a pickup speeding parallel to the train. Apparently, there had been a miscommunication—they used flags or lanterns, not radio, to signal—and the engineer, who rode at the front of the train, had left the conductor, who rode in the caboose, standing on the station platform. The truck, conductor in tow, was racing to catch up.

A few stops after the conductor got on the train, we pulled into the Memphis station just as the sun was setting. I stuffed—and I do mean stuffed—my seabag and the manila envelope with my records and transfer papers into a train station locker, then turned around and bumped the bag with my butt to get the door closed.

My rumbling belly urged me in the direction of downtown, where I could rustle up some dinner. The jazzy notes of trombone, piano, and drums floated out along the cool evening breeze, and I felt a pull toward the music. I loved jazz. When I'd learned that I was being transferred to Millington, a city just outside of Memphis, I'd put Beale Street on my to-do list. *Here I am!* I thought. *Home of the blues.* It was Saturday night, and the sidewalks teemed with people, mostly Black. (Perhaps one of the other white people was a young Elvis Presley, who was a year my junior, on break from his job at nearby Loews Theater—he often visited Beale Street for the same reason I was there.) I weaved my way through, tipping my hat at ladies of a certain age, inhaling the spicy-sweet scent of barbecue. My mouth watered as I weighed the pros and cons of a pulled-pork sandwich versus slow-smoked ribs.

I was awakened from my contemplations when a shore patrol paddy wagon pulled up next to me. "Sailor," said the petty officer in the passenger seat, "what are you doing on Beale Street?"

"Looking for a place to eat and some live jazz, sir."

"You are off-limits. Let me see your liberty card."

"I don't have a liberty card," I said. "I've been transferred to Millington, and I haven't checked into the base yet, so I'm still on leave."

"Let me see your transfer papers, then."

"They're in a locker with my seabag at the train station."

The shore patrol petty officer told me to get in. "We'll go on a little drive down to the train station, take a look at those transfer papers," he said.

I reluctantly opened the back door and slid onto the back seat. For the short trip, we rode in silence. At the station, it took me a minute to open the locker door because of the pressure of my seabag pushing against it. I had to lean hard into the door to turn the key, and when I finally managed to get the key turned, the door flew open with a clang. "Here," I said, adding "sir" as I handed over my papers.

The SP shuffled through them and, satisfied, let me know that they were not going to take me in. "Just don't let us catch you on Beale Street again, you hear?" the officer said. I nodded. "Where're you staying for the night?"

"I am going to find a YMCA."

The two men looked at each other, and the man who'd been driving the paddy wagon shrugged. "Our watch is over at midnight," he said. "We can take you to the base with us then if you want."

"How am I going to get on the base and sign in so late? I thought I had to wait till after 08:00."

"That's easy. When we get to the gate, we'll tell the jarhead on guard duty that we are taking you to the brig, and they'll wave us through. We can find you a bed at the brig even if you have to sleep in an empty cell."

"What about my stuff?" I said, gesturing to my seabag.

"In the morning, have breakfast, come back and get your seabag and papers, and check in."

"Sounds good to me."

"Be standing at the curb in front of the station at 24:00." The driver checked his watch. "Make that 23:50 in case we are early."

I was sad about missing my chance to visit Beale Street, but I did as told and wandered down to the docks and ate a dinner of catfish pulled fresh from the Mississippi River that morning. The temperature dropped as November's early darkness fell, and so I walked along Riverside Drive and then up to Main Street and Front Street to stay warm. There was plenty to see, and I could enjoy the blues and jazz from a distance.

I returned to the station at 23:50, my belly full and my legs pleasantly tired. The two patrolmen pulled up and I got in. "You know," said the petty officer on the passenger side, looking over his left shoulder toward me in the back seat, "the next time you're on Beale Street, make sure that you're wearing civilian clothes."

"Those polished black navy shoes are a dead giveaway," the driver added. "Buy yourself a pair of brown penny loafers."

"Yeah, and twenty-year-olds wearing all-new clothes look suspicious to us. I'd recommend going to a thrift store like Goodwill."

At the base, we were waved through, and they found me an actual bed. I was a little disappointed—I would have liked to be able to say that I'd spent a night in the brig—but I was glad when my head hit the pillow.

LIFE ON BASE

World War I was the first war in which aircraft were used as weaponry. The fighting was going on way across the pond in Europe, but the American government feared that we might be dragged into the conflict, and so Park Field, a World War I training base for the army's signal corps, was built in Millington, Tennessee, in 1917. The Aviation Section had 1,218 men and 280 aircraft.

The airplane used for training army pilots was the Curtiss JN series biplane, or Jenny. At the end of the war, in 1918, the US Postal Service began using the Jenny for delivering airmail, and after the war, the army sold off surplus supplies, including Jennys. At around $500 apiece—the annual average salary in 1918 was $1,500—in combination with zero government aviation regulations, this clearance sale gave birth to "barnstorming," in which touring acrobats traveled to rural areas to put on air shows. Flying circuses drew huge crowds of ticket-buying customers. Stunt fliers surpassed vaudeville stars in their popularity, but acrobatics at high speeds hundreds of feet in the air is a lot more dangerous. Barnstormers did handstands on the wings, flew suicidally low to the ground, swung on ropes from aircraft to aircraft. Any mistake or miscalculation could be, and was, fatal.

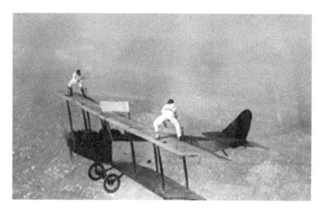

Playing tennis on the wing of a Curtiss Jenny, 1925

Japan attacked Pearl Harbor on December 7, 1941. The United States declared war against Japan the next day, and three days later, Germany declared war against us. War on two fronts—in Europe and in the South Pacific—meant a reinvestment in air warfare, and on January 1, 1943, Park Field was renamed Naval Air Station Memphis and the training base was designated the Naval Air Technical Training Center.

When I arrived at the naval air station on November 23, 1952, I joined approximately thirteen thousand uniformed and civilian naval personnel. I checked in at 08:00 Sunday morning, one day early, with Petty Officer Brodie, who was in charge of our barracks. "There are going to be ten in your class," he told me, showing me a diagram of the sleeping quarters. "You'll be sharing the first five bunks on the port side. You're the third in your class to check in so far, and I recommend the top bed of this bunk"—he pointed to the bunk next to the window in the first cubicle—"because the bottom beds always become couches for the cubicle, and the guy in the top bunk will wake you while climbing up if he goes to bed later than you."

"Sounds good to me. Which locker goes with it?"

He pointed to the one next to the wall.

"I expected more of my classmates to be here already," I said. "The other seven are cutting it close."

"They're in the OGU. They'll be here tomorrow."

"What's the OGU?"

"You've never been in the outgoing unit? Lucky you. It's a unit of transient sailors waiting for class to start or to receive travel orders to the next duty station. They get the bottom-of-the-food-chain duties while they're waiting. How have you been able to avoid it?"

"After boot camp, my leave was cut short because of the starting date of ANP school, and there were less than two weeks between my going from Norman to here. I took another leave because I knew I'd be gone for six months. I still have a little over a week of leave on the books for this year."

"You'll probably get introduced when you finish TD school. We'll want you out of the barracks to make room for the next incoming class."

At just before 10:00, the group of seven showed up. The barracks was empty because the advanced students sharing the space had marched off to class at 08:00. Brodie lined us up, and we got the rules and regulations of life under his command. He pointed out the directions to the head (what civilians call "the toilet"), the showers, water basins, laundry room, and study area. Last, he pointed out the three cubicles our class would occupy. "A bottom bunk is available in the first cubicle, the other two cubicles are open on a first-come-first-served basis. I'll be back in fifteen minutes to record where you are going to be living the next twenty-two weeks."

Conversation broke out as soon as Petty Officer Brodie headed to his office. One member of the class stepped out of line and walked over to my cubicle with a "Hey! Bryce, huh? You from Gila Valley?"

The first thing that entered my mind was: *How did he know my name?* Then it dawned on me that my name was over my shirt pocket. "I was born there but moved when I was a kid. My mom and dad were from Ashurst."

"I'm from Glenbar. We must be related."

"Larson doesn't ring a bell," I said, checking the name over his shirt pocket. "But I was five the last time I lived in Ashurst."

"Mind if I join you?"

"If you don't mind the bottom bunk, you are more than welcome."

It turned out that Clay Larson and I were second cousins. His mother and my paternal grandfather were brother and sister. We became close friends, closer than any other sailor I served with.

The next morning, we lined up with the other classes, and at 08:00, we marched to class. The morning was typical navy: roll call, more rules, more regulations, and orientation. Next came the class syllabus: math, physics, electronics, Link Trainer operation and maintenance, movie projector operation and maintenance. All were subjects I was glad to study.

Life on base was pretty mundane and repetitive. Every fourth day, I'd have night watch duty, which, I quickly realized, was pointless. I can remember standing at midnight outside the school area, watching the old, unused World War II munition bunkers with rusted doors while rain poured down and the temperature dropped below forty degrees. I carried a Springfield M1 rifle that had the barrel plugged and the firing pin removed, no ammunition, and, anyway, I and everything else was soaking wet. My main job was to monitor the road that was a back way to officer housing. Whenever a car approached, I checked the officer decal on the lower left corner of the windshield, saluted, and waved them through. I thought, *I*

*don't know him in uniform or civilian clothing, I just salute and
wave. He could be a thief and I would have no idea.*

When I tried to explain to the watch petty officer how stupid the watch and guarding empty bunkers was and the use-
lessness of a gun with a plugged barrel and no firing pin, for
four hours in pneumonia weather, I got rewarded by getting
the midnight watch out at the munition bunkers every watch
day until he got transferred about two months later.

JIM CROW IS NOT IN THE GOOD BOOK

That wasn't the only instance of sheer stupidity I'd encounter
during my time in the South. Not to say it was all bad. While
on leave, buddies and I would hitchhike to wherever the person
who picked us up was going. One of my favorites was the Sam
D. Hamilton Noxubee National Wildlife Refuge in Mississippi,
just south of Starkville. We spent most of the day canoeing in
a swampy area that had a grove of cypress trees growing right
out of the water, watching for beavers, muskrats, nutria, and,
of course, alligators. Wood ducks and Canada geese floated
alongside our little canoe while red-cockaded woodpeckers
knocked on trees along the shore. White-tailed deer, gray and
fox squirrels, and rabbits skirted the cottonmouth, copper-
head, timber, and pygmy rattlesnakes that were rumored to
slink within the underbrush. It was a moment of peace amid
the monotony.

I also loved Hot Springs National Park in Arkansas, though
we couldn't afford the cost of a meal or lodging in the area.
I took my freedom of movement for granted—until a friend
and I were picked up by a middle-aged Black man heading to
Mississippi. An hour into the ride, he took out a little green
book from his glove box and handed it to me. "Can you flip
through and find a nearby gas station in there?" he asked.

"We just passed a gas station," I said. "Why don't we turn around? Won't take but a minute."

The man glanced over at us, a couple of blond, blue-eyed, clean-cut white boys. "I'm not welcome at that gas station," he said. "If I were to pull over and let my dog out on the side of the road to pee, no one would think twice. But if I did the same, the police would have me in handcuffs fast as you please. That book is a guidebook for Black people in this area—where it's safe to get gas, go to the bathroom, grab a bite to eat, that sort of thing."

I was surprised, though I shouldn't have been. It wasn't like I'd never seen bigotry and its destructiveness, the pain it causes, before. My earliest memory of racism was when I was in the fourth grade and, one day, my good friend Hana simply disappeared. When I asked my teacher where Hana was, she answered, "We are at war with Japan. Hana's family is Japanese . . ."

"So?" I asked.

The teacher sighed. "Well, they could be helping our enemy. So they've been taken to live in a camp for a little while, just so we can keep an eye on them."

I mulled over her answer for a minute. "But we're also at war with Germany, aren't we? So why are the German kids still here?"

There was a long, deafening silence. "It's recess," she finally said, nodding toward the window and the view of kids running and jumping rope outside. "Go and play."

When I got home, I asked Mom the same question. "German people look like us," she told me. "It would be harder to figure out who is from Germany." To my ten-year-old ears, this sounded ridiculous, but she seemed satisfied with her answer.

The federal government would incarcerate a hundred and twenty thousand people of Japanese ancestry, including seventeen thousand children under the age of ten, and force them to relocate to internment camps. And that was that.

A few years later, a Black high school in my area burned down. In segregated Arizona, school districts had the option to choose to be integrated—and most passed. (*Brown v. Board of Education* wouldn't rule "separate but equal" unconstitutional until 1954.) Most stayed firm in their choice, even after the fire made it so all those Black kids had nowhere to go to school. My school, Mesa High, was the exception. There was an adjustment period, sure, but soon enough, everyone got used to it. And then there was Chaffee High and Compton High in California, where I lived during my sophomore and senior years. They were integrated, too.

So, though I'd certainly been around bigotry, the racism in Tennessee and its neighboring states was like nothing I'd ever seen before. Ninety years after the Civil War, the racial segregation enforced by the Jim Crow laws, so named after a blackface character in minstrel theater, was in full swing. Ku Klux Klan membership was at a low (a state of affairs that would soon change as the civil rights movement ramped up), but people didn't need white robes and funny hats to oppress Black people with the threat of violence, or actual violence. There had been 236 lynchings in Tennessee alone from 1877 to 1950, a number that only accounted for those on record; in the nation, mostly in the South, there were more than 4,000. This was no distant memory in 1952 but a real threat and reasonable fear for Black people, and even on city streets, the atmosphere buzzed with tension.

I soon realized that my little visit to Beale Street was not without its dangers—not for me, as a white sailor on his way to base, but for those I interacted with. Grandma Herbert had instilled in me the Golden Rule, to do unto others as you would have them do unto you, which I took at face value. And so I had walked down Beale Street tipping my hat indiscriminately, oblivious to the fact that Black pedestrians were quick to avert their eyes and get out of my way.

BEFORE ROSA PARKS

Three years before Rosa Parks went to jail for refusing to give up her seat to a white man in Montgomery, Alabama, the city bus was a venue in which racism often played out. Cities couldn't afford a whites-only bus and a Blacks-only bus, so the races were forced to mingle—or, rather, white people were forced to mingle with Black people—often with explosive results.

One afternoon, I was heading into town to have Sunday dinner with the family of a young woman I'd met at a USO dance, when I happened to sit by an older white woman in a church dress and hat. Back then, we didn't think twice about commenting on a woman's appearance, and so I said, "What a pretty hat you're wearing."

She smiled. "I try to wear my finest to church to show my respect for God," she said. "We had a lovely sermon today about how God made man in his own image, and it is our responsibility to be more like him in our spiritual, moral, and intellectual nature." I nodded amicably. After a few seconds, she blurted out, "Do you believe in evolution?"

"Yes, I do," I said, taken aback.

And then she preceded to go on the most racist rant I'd ever heard.

Being a nineteen-year-old aspiring scientist, I attempted to reconcile the God she'd spoken of with the science as I knew it. "Evolution is how God created *all living things* on Earth," I said, emphasizing "all living things" as a way to gently push back against her sense of superiority.

"No," she said, shaking her head sadly. "It's in the Bible.

God created us white folks in his own image out of the dust of the earth, six thousand years ago."

That was the end of the conversation. I'd learned a valuable lesson: It is very difficult, if not impossible, to reason with hate-fueled nonsense. Especially when it is reinforced by an authority, like the church, or when it benefits those in power, or makes people feel better about themselves through tearing down others.

A couple weeks later, on my way to a USO dance, I boarded a Memphis city bus to find that there was only one seat left, an aisle seat just in front of the four-inch painted white line on the floor, sides, and ceiling just behind the second bus door. The line separated the Black section at the back from the white section in front. The Black passengers were packed in like sardines.

After a couple of stops, a pregnant Black woman boarded, an infant on one hip and a sack of groceries on the other. The driver didn't wait until she was seated before pulling out onto the road, and she stumbled down the aisle. I automatically put my hand on her arm to help steady her, my grandmother's indoctrination kicking in, plus the old-fashioned sense of chivalry my dad had imparted. I could practically hear him saying, *Always offer your seat to a woman, especially if she is pregnant.* I jumped up without thinking and said, "Here, have my seat."

All hell broke loose. The woman who had been sitting next to me, said, a look of utter disgust on her face, "I don't want no n— sitting next to me."

Again, without thinking, I replied, "In that case, get on up. She and her baby need those seats more than we do."

From the front of the bus came the shout "You damn n— lover!"

From the back of the bus came the loud reply "I stick the first man that touches him!"

The bus came to a screeching stop in the middle of the street and the back door flew open. "Out!" yelled the bus driver. The young lady almost fell again as she rushed to get behind the white line; I disembarked before she caught my trouble.

The bus pulled away with a roar, leaving me on an unfamiliar street, scratching my head and looking for the next bus stop.

POKING THE BEAR

Still, my head is nothing if not hard, and I couldn't always stop myself from poking the bear. Or, if not poking the bear, then ignoring the bear. Because the bear was an idiot.

Often, I'd spend the day before a USO dance wandering around downtown Memphis, enjoying my time away from the base without any agenda. One afternoon, I spotted a Woolworth's and decided to get a soda at the lunch counter. All the seats were taken, and a few people were waiting for an open seat. I didn't feel like hanging around for a soda, so I figured I'd just get a drink of water. There were two drinking fountains, one with a sign over it that read "Whites Only" and one with the sign "Colored Only." The one designated for whites had a line of five or six people, while the other was unoccupied. So I did what I thought was the sensible thing and got a drink of water at the empty fountain. The water relieved my parched throat, and I sighed with relief. But when I finished and turned around, there stood two white men. "Can't you read?" one of them said. "That fountain is for n— only."

Gesturing over my left shoulder to the sign, I answered, "No, it says 'Colored Only,' and I'm a light tan color."

The other guy said, "You smart-ass Yankee. You're leaving this store right now." Then they each grabbed an arm and escorted me to the front door and out onto the sidewalk.

All the while—and I can't believe I did this, now that I'm writing it—I offered a lesson on plumbing, on how one pipe delivers the water to a tee, which sends that same water to both fountains. So, really, what's the point?

"We better not see your sorry face in here again," said the first guy.

A month or two later, I was attending an LDS meeting when James, a member of the base personnel rather than a student, showed up. He owned a 1941 four-door Cadillac sedan and, more importantly, had a list of single Southern girls he'd met while on his mission in Louisiana and Arkansas.

James invited three of us to take a four-hour road trip to meet some girls in Pine Bluff, Arkansas. On the way, we stopped for lunch at a roadside hamburger stand. James pulled up and parked in the available space next to the "Colored Only" window. "I'll get it," I volunteered. "Four burgers, four fries, and four sodas," I said, smiling at the Black gal at the window. I paid and waited for her to bring the soft drinks. "It'll be just a few minutes," she said, looking wary.

I took the sodas to my pals, then leaned back against the back passenger-side door. The day was cool, and I pulled my collar up around my neck. After a few minutes, the woman called out, "Your burgers are ready," and so I approached the window and took the paper bag, the scent of French fries making my mouth water. "Thanks," I said. Just then, a pack of high school boys rounded the corner.

"That window is for colored only," one of them yelled. "You can't eat those!"

"They were cooked on the same grill as your burgers were," I replied, acting nonchalant while picking up my pace to the car. The engine roared to life.

One of the boys came up to me and grabbed my shoulder. "What are you, some kind of freak!"

With his touch and tone, I got a shot of adrenaline and

survival mode kicked in—in this case, it was the "fight" part of "fight, flight, or freeze." I stomped on his foot, and he let go, his head dropping just enough to become a perfect target. I swung around and clocked him with the side of my fist; he dropped to the ground. The other boys started running toward me, and I took off running, and as I got to the car, the back door swung open. (I didn't know if James was more worried about me or his car.) I tossed the bag of burgers in the back seat and dived in behind them.

We rode in silence for a minute before my friend Arnold, who was sitting on the other side of the back seat, picked up the paper bag. "These smell good," he said, passing out our lunch, "you damn fool."

I shrugged. "I guess we shouldn't stop there on the way back," I said, unwrapping my burger.

BLOOD IS RED

Word got around that a local girl was going to have an operation and might need a large quantity of blood, and there was a call for donors at the base. I volunteered because my type O negative blood was the universal donor. The navy provided a bus to take us to the hospital in Memphis, and when we got there, I learned that they already had enough, that my donation was not needed. I had some time to kill before the bus returned us to base, and I was wandering around outside when an ambulance pulled up to the entrance of the emergency room. I stood still, watching the drama from a safe distance. The medics jumped out the back and rolled out the gurney, which held a Black man, his face slack and the sheet over him stained a bright, gory crimson. Once they were inside, the driver of the ambulance parked and got out. "My, that sheet was redder than it was white," I said. "He's going to need a lot of blood."

"Yeah, he was in a fight and got knifed a bunch of times. He's lost a lot of blood, he's lucky to be alive."

"Turns out I was brought down here by the navy to give blood for a little girl who's having an operation, but she doesn't need mine. I'm O negative, I'd be happy to donate blood for that man if he needs it."

The driver stopped and looked at me. "First off, it doesn't work that way," he said, irritation in his voice. "They take blood from the blood bank, not as a direct transfer. Second, we don't give white blood to n—."

That ruffled my feathers. "Last time I checked," I said, "all blood is red."

CHAPTER 4

Litchfield Naval Air

After tradevman school, I rode the train fifteen hundred miles west to Goodyear, Arizona, to start work at Litchfield Park Naval Air Facility. I'd lived there not so long before, during fourth, fifth, and sixth grades, when my dad worked first as a contractor for the company in charge of building new homes for the incoming wartime workforce, then as a welder for the Goodyear Aircraft factory. My pregnant mom and my dad bought one of the federally funded 750-square-foot houses, and they moved in, along with me, my sister, my aunt Falene, her baby Jearldene, my uncle Talmage, my cousin Milton Junior, and their friend Joe Brown. The town was undeveloped back then, but I found a way to keep myself—and my poor beleaguered parents—busy, breaking my arm on the monkey bars, setting a field full of old Christmas trees on fire, buying a (possibly stolen) donkey for two dollars, getting rattled out of a giant cottonwood tree by a plane passing overhead. It was in Goodyear that I discovered my all-time favorite science teacher, Mr. Kühn, in whose footsteps I hoped to follow.

After World War II ended, the navy took control of the Goodyear Aircraft Corporation's 8,500-foot runway and the 789 acres adjacent to the factory. The area's warm, dry climate was ideal for storage, and our primary function was to "mothball" the navy, marine, and coast guard airplanes that were no longer needed. At one point, the grounds hosted more than 5,000 aircraft.

The base itself was small and had less than ten pilots to ferry in the aircraft, as well as approximately 150 naval personnel in other support roles. There were also a number of civil servants—including my uncle Bill, my dad's second-youngest brother—who prepared the planes for storage. I had been transferred to LPNAF to unpack a Link Trainer from its shipping crates, set it up, and operate it to help the pilots keep their instrument flying certification up to date.

The Link Trainer was invented by Edwin Albert Link, who took his first flying lesson in 1920, at the age of sixteen. Ed had a passion for flying but couldn't afford the cost of lessons, so he decided to build something that would allow him to practice on his own. Using the technology and his knowledge of bellows, valves, and pumps gained from working in his father's piano and organ factory, he started an eighteen-month project to develop an on-the-ground simulator, which was driven by an electric pump to pitch and roll as the pilot worked the controls.

Ed founded the Link Aeronautical Corporation in 1929, selling most of his Link Trainers as carnival rides at amusement parks. But then, in 1934, the Army Air Corps took over transporting US airmail, and in a seventy-eight-day period, twelve pilots were killed because of their inability to read the instruments during poor conditions or at night. This loss prompted the Air Corps to reconsider the Link Trainer, and the deal was clinched when Ed Link flew through a fogbank previously regarded as unflyable. The Air Corps bought six Link Trainers to start.

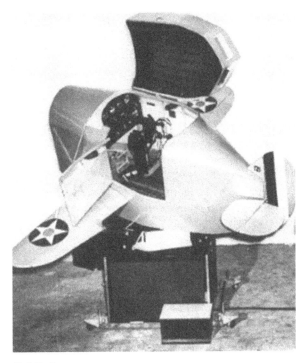

Link Trainer

Learning how to maintain and repair a Link Trainer would eventually come in handy. Years later, my eldest daughter, Vicki, at the age of eight, decided she wanted to learn how to play the piano. Her mother found an advertisement in the paper that announced that the Mayflower moving company was selling unclaimed storage items. She called to see if there was a piano. "Looks like there's a player piano," the guy on the line told her, "but the player component doesn't work. The keyboard works fine, just needs tuning."

"How much?" Joyce asked.

"Just the storage debt of ninety dollars. We'll throw in three boxes of player rolls while we're at it." It was a steal, a true antique. I was easily able to make the repairs, then I used a couple coats of dark Old English and some varnish to make the wood surface look like new.

But in the spring of 1953, when I inquired about where to get the necessary tools to uncrate the trainer, a rebellion broke out. The pilots were being certified at Naval Air Station North Island, and opening an instrument certification operation on our base would mean no trip to San Diego, no two or three days off duty, no lying on the beach and all that with per diem. Needless to say, I lost that battle.

Without a Link Trainer, I had no job. I am not one to just sit around, so, out of sheer boredom, I approached Personnel to see about getting transferred. "We'll need a few days to get something lined up," the yeoman on duty said, examining me over the top of his bifocals. A few days later, he called me in to tell me to report to the chief petty officer (CPO) in charge of recreation. For two weeks, I maintained the softball field, which was never played on, at least not while I was there.

I am also not one to be satisfied doing busywork. Thanks to the captain's wife, however, I got a new job—the captain's yeoman had phoned the CPO to let him know that the captain and his wife wanted to host twenty friends for a private show-ing of *Roman Holiday* a week from Saturday. The next day, the CPO called me into his office and told me, "I had no idea how I was going to get a projectionist in time. The manual says that it takes a tradevman, and since you're the only tradevman on base, you get the job. Lucky you."

"You gotta be kidding!" I said, raising my eyebrows. "I was trained on sixteen-millimeter projectors, sir, not a thirty-five millimeter. I've seen pictures of a thirty-five-millimeter projector but have never seen one in real life, let alone operated one."

"I guess you have a lot to learn in not a lot of time. Here's the keys to the booth." He tossed me the keys, which I caught one-handed. "I'll assign a work party to get the theater ready," he added. He nodded to excuse me, then held up a finger as though remembering something. "Oh, and you'll need to procure the movie."

"How do I do that?"

"I hear you're no dummy. You'll figure it out." And with that, I was excused.

The outdoor theater had a professional screen with a box frame and room for about fifty people. Eight-foot-long benches with backs made up rows; only the front four rows had waterproof plastic cushions for the officers. The theater hadn't been used in weeks, for good reason: the temperature at sunset was approximately a hundred degrees, and even with two big fans, it would be uncomfortable. I scanned the seats, shielding my face from the sun's glare with my hand and noting the layer of dust, spotted here and there with bird droppings. *This is going to need a thorough scrubbing,* I thought with a sigh.

I climbed the steps to the projection booth. Inside were two thirty-five-millimeter carbon-arc projectors and, in a drawer of a filing cabinet, the manual. I flipped through the pages. I already was somewhat familiar with a carbon arc light—two carbon electrode rods of different electric polarities strike each other to ignite the rods, which are then slowly separated. This increases the temperature until it reaches the vaporization point of the carbon at approximately 6,600 degrees Fahrenheit, producing an extremely bright white light. You must stop there or the arc will go out; there is a mechanism in the lamp that controls the gap size as the carbon burns to prevent the light from going out.

The manual was a big help but not big enough. I soon learned that a single reel of a thousand feet of film moves through the projector at twenty-four frames per second, meaning one reel takes approximately eleven minutes, and therefore an average movie would be nine or ten reels. On top of that, I'd have to master the cue marks in order to not stall the movie between reels. Tiny white dots in the upper-right-hand corner of the film signaled that the reel was ending. The first cue, the motor cue, came eight seconds before the end of the reel and meant it was time to turn on the second projector. The next cue, the changeover cue, was one second before the end and meant it was time to turn on the run switch. Each mark lasted for four frames, or 0.17 seconds, and it took a little while to learn how to spot them. (Once you can see them, however, you can't unsee them. Until the industry started switching from film to digital in the early 2000s, I could never watch a movie without being aware of the cues.)

I was in way over my head. I convinced the chief to arrange for me to observe Carl, the projectionist at the Luke Air Force Base five miles north of us. Folks were clearly smarter at Luke AFB: they had an air-conditioned theater, and Carl was a full-time nonmilitary projectionist. First I observed him, then he observed me to make sure I had the hang of it, and he helped me locate the film. I was surprised when it came; it was eleven reels.

The captain's wife's social event went off without a hitch. Well, at least the movie ran smoothly, though the guests quickly wilted in the heat. We had the movie for another week, so the CPO asked me to show it every night for the sailors and personnel. It had three strikes against it: one, the temperature was one-hundred-plus degrees; two, the rom-com *Roman Holiday*, even with Audrey Hepburn as its star, was not exactly made for the eighteen-to-twenty-year-old male demographic; three, there was no concession stand. Only a few people showed up, and I ended up shutting down the operation after the third night. (It reopened on the cooler night of October 10, and they hired a nonmilitary projectionist.)

I had another meeting with the CPO about my assignments. "It's too damn hot for watching movies outside or playing softball," I said. "Can I be transferred to a base that actually needs a tradevman?"

He gave me the same answer. "I need a few days to work something out," then added, "You can return the film and clean up the projection booth while you're waiting."

"It's clean. The circuit breakers and the master switch are turned off. I put in a new set of carbon rods, the film is boxed and ready to be picked up, and the door is locked."

"Huh," he said, squinting at me. After a moment, he asked, "Don't your folks live in the LA area?"

"Yes, sir, in Compton."

"After the film is picked up tomorrow, go ahead and take off and visit your folks. I'll file for basket leave"—paperwork for an informal leave, which, if nothing happens to the sailor while gone, gets torn up and thrown in the wastebasket once he returns—"and I'll see you Monday morning at 08:00. I'll have a new job for you by then."

JUST ANOTHER DAY AT THE OFFICE

My family was surprised to see me, and my mom baked me a couple of my favorite lemon meringue pies over the weekend. When I walked into the chief's office Monday morning, he greeted me with "Do you know how to swim?"

"Yes," I said, already leery. "Why do you want to know?"

"We need another lifeguard. I assume you don't have a valid lifeguard certificate?" I nodded. "Fine. I booked you for a three-day Red Cross certificate training that starts on Wednesday morning at the Y. Come on, let's go over to the pool and I'll introduce you to the lifeguards on duty. Larry and Glenn'll show you the ropes."

The next Monday morning, I showed up an hour early for the crew meeting with a certificate and two new bathing suits in hand. It was already hot, and the bright blue of the pool looked inviting.

"All right," said the chief. "Let's get our assignments straight for the week."

Larry, who was the oldest at around thirty, had dark circles under his eyes and a grumpy expression on his face. "I'm not a morning person," he said with gravel in his voice.

"I am," I said. "I can take the early shift."

Glenn and the fourth lifeguard, Jeff, both in their late twenties, were also night people. "One of you is going to have to take the early shift when you're on duty," the chief said. "You guys decide, I don't care. How about you two teams take turns every other day?"

"We'll never get a weekend off with that schedule," Larry said.

"We could do two on and two off," said Glenn.

I piped up, "That would give us a weekend every four weeks. To get the weekend off every other week, we'll need to make it a three-day weekend. Two days on, two days off, three days on, two days off, two days on, three days off, will repeat every two weeks. So, we will get a three-day weekend off every other week."

"Sound good to me," the chief said with a shrug. "Let's do it."

I didn't bring up the fact that we would be working two days one week and five the next. Larry and I started that very morning, which meant that I'd be on duty the first weekend.

The pool was open to personnel and their families. All navy personnel had to pass swimming in boot camp for obvious reasons—if the ship goes down or you fall overboard, you better be able to swim. I wasn't worried much about them, but their kids were a different matter, and a young boy named Tommy, in particular. His twenty-seven-year-old mom was there to sunbathe, not to watch her son. She must have thought that was what the lifeguards were for. As soon as they arrived, before she'd even unpacked their towels, she would tell Tommy, "You do what the lifeguards tell you to do." Then she'd start rubbing her homemade suntan lotion of baby oil and tincture of iodine over her skin. She asked me more than once if I would apply it to her back—apparently, that was another thing lifeguards were for. Don't get me wrong, I didn't exactly mind. But I didn't like the telltale dark stain the iodine left on my hands. Once oiled up, she would lay down on her beach towel. Every twenty to thirty minutes, I'd have to remind her to turn over so she wouldn't get sunburned.

I liked Tommy. He kind of reminded me of me when I was his age, in that he wasn't so much a troublemaker as he was a fun seeker, a boundary pusher, a risk-taker. He knew he could get away with more when Mom wasn't watching, and he was afraid of nothing. I'd try to keep him in the shallow end of the pool, but he'd find a way to get in water over his head. He couldn't swim but kept his nose above the water by thrashing his arms and legs. Then, when he got tired, he'd start yelling for help, confident that I would come to the rescue. It became a game with him. He would climb up the three-meter tower and jump off, then thrash around until I jumped in and let him hang on my back while I towed him to the shallow end. After two days of that, I decided it was time to teach him to swim. It didn't take very long. I made a game out of it, telling him, "Tip your right shoulder and reach your right arm under the water in front of you, then cup your hand and pull as much of the water as you can behind you. Then do the same with your left. Move your feet up and down so the fish can't bite your toes!" Like many kids, he didn't like to put his face in the water, so, to motivate him, I scattered a handful of pennies on the bottom of the shallow end. "You can keep the ones you pick up," I said.

That got him moving. The chief got word of me giving Tommy swim lessons and talked me into teaching a class open to all personnel kids. It cost me a lot of pennies, but it was worth it.

DOUBLE TROUBLE

To cater to Larry's hatred of mornings, he and I split the day. I worked from 08:00 to 15:00, and his shift went from 12:30 to 19:30. I did the routine chlorine and pH tests and made any necessary adjustments, washed the decks, opened the restrooms and checked to see if they needed any supplies. Then I unlocked the gate.

I met two teenagers, Carolyn and Suzy, on my very first day. On my third duty day, I went to unlock the gate to find Suzy already there waiting to get in. "Good morning," I said with a smile. She smiled at me, then headed to the women's dressing room. I surveyed the deck one more time, then took a seat on the lifeguard's chair. A few minutes later, I heard someone approach and turned to see Suzy standing there in her two-piece bathing suit (the word "bikini" wasn't well known in the United States yet, and wouldn't be for another decade or so), holding the unfastened top over her breasts with her left arm. "Would you mind fastening my straps in the back?" she asked.

Sometimes nineteen-year-olds do stupid things, and I do mean stupid! "Sure," I said, climbing down from the tower. And I did. "Thanks," she said, rubbing her hand across the back of my shoulders before jumping into the pool. The splash woke me up. *What the hell were you thinking?* I thought. *Do you have a brain in your head?* Then I saw the red flags waving all around me.

The next morning, Suzy did it again. This time, I refused. "You'll need to return to the dressing room and not come out until you are properly dressed," I told her, looking away when she pursed her lips into a pout. "I'm sorry, but, otherwise, I will have to bar you from using the pool." She must have taken me seriously because the next day she was properly dressed. But that didn't stop her from flirting with me.

"I have a very jealous wife," I finally lied to deter her.

I turned and there was Suzy's friend Carolyn, who was just arriving, her bag and a towel tucked under her arm. "I didn't know you were married," she said. "You're not wearing a ring."

"Yeah, sure, I have three wives," I replied, upping the ante. "They live in Short Creek."

The teenage girls looked at each other. Even non-Mormons knew about Short Creek, the polygamist Mormon town on the Utah-Arizona border. Six years earlier, in 1947, Arizona's governor had initiated a raid on the community. It's difficult to arrive unannounced in the desert, however, and when the townspeople saw a great cloud of dust on the road leading into town, the men fled and the women stood in a line to greet the police, singing hymns. All wives but the first were not recognized as legal by the state, a blessing for young girls who'd been forced into marriage or those with abusive husbands, but for those who were content with their lot as second or third wives, this was more of a headache than anything. They would leave for a while, only to return when the dust settled.

"I don't believe you have three wives at Short Creek," Suzy said.

Larry must have caught part of that conversation because later he asked if he could give me some advice. "I noticed that you've been flirting with a couple of the girls. Carolyn is seventeen, and she's the exec's daughter. You're a white hat"—slang for an enlisted sailor below chief—"need I remind you. And Suzy is a chief's daughter, and she is only *fifteen*. She's got a case of hormones, which spells big trouble. Be careful."

SOMEONE TATTLED

I had a life-changing liberty from Friday, July 24, through Sunday, July 26, 1953. On Friday, I met my wife-to-be. On Saturday, we had our first date. (More on that later.)

On Sunday, I got bit on the butt but didn't know it till Monday morning. I was whistling a jaunty tune when I pulled up to the front gate at 07:00. "You are to report to the exec's office at 08:30," the guard told me. From his tone of voice, I knew I'd better use the next hour and a half to shine my shoes, brush off my blues, and put on a clean hat. *Did he hear I was flirting with his daughter?* I wondered nervously.

At 08:30 on the dot, I rapped my knuckles on the exec's office door. "Come in," came a gruff voice from inside. I walked in and saluted. "Have a seat," the large, ruddy-faced man behind the desk said. The exec was wearing the summer uniform of a short-sleeve khaki shirt with a gold maple leaf on each collar to show his rank, a chest loaded with ribbons, and his hair combed neatly to the side. I sat down on one of the two visitor chairs and realized that the other one was occupied. "This is Mr. Crawford, state public safety officer," the exec said, gesturing to the man in similar attire next to me. Though Mr. Crawford had an office job, it was clear that he spent time outside, perhaps playing sports or working on a farm. "He has some questions for you."

I extended my hand to shake, perplexed. "At your service, sir," I said.

He shook my hand, then cleared his throat. "What do you know about Short Creek, and where did you get your information?"

I leaned back in my chair, still perplexed. "I've known about Short Creek since I was a kid, sir. When I was a freshman in high school, my grandfather married a woman named

Eva Spencer who had left the Mormon Fundamentalist Church there and was living with her sister in Mesa."

There was a pause as Mr. Crawford wrote down my answer. Then he looked sharply at me. "Tell me who you know that lives in or has ties to Short Creek."

"I don't know anyone other than Eva, and I only know her because she was married to my grandfather in 1947. She had to leave during that raid. But they were married for a very short time. I have no idea where she is now."

On the word "raid," Mr. Crawford's ears seemed to perk up. "When did you know about the raid?" he asked.

"When it happened . . . in 1947."

Mr. Crawford sighed. "No, not that raid. The raid yesterday morning."

"I, uh, I'm not sure what you're talking about. I don't know anything about a raid."

"The raid on Short Creek yesterday morning," Mr. Crawford said slowly, as though I were new to the English language. "It's been on the news all day long, since yesterday morning."

I shook my head. "As I said, I don't know anything about a raid. I was in California on liberty this weekend and got back to the base this morning."

"My daughter told me that you said you have three wives living in Short Creek," the exec said. "We can't find anything in your records about you being married."

I almost smiled but stopped myself. "Sir, there isn't anything there, because I'm not married and never have been. I was just joking."

The safety officer scowled. "Someone tipped off Short Creek that we were coming."

I looked back and forth between the exec and Mr. Crawford. "Surely, you know that wasn't me?"

"It's a little odd, you mentioning Short Creek just days be-fore the raid, don't you think?" said the exec. "When the news hit, I tried to get ahold of you, but I was told you were on lib-erty, and they didn't know where you were. I thought if you had three wives there, state officials might be interested in talking with you, so I called the National Guard." He shrugged.

"Well, I do not have three wives, I do not have any wives, and no one I know besides my grandpa's ex-wife ever lived in Short Creek."

Mr. Crawford closed his notebook and said, "I think I have all the information I need for now. You might be called to tes-tify, so don't be surprised if you hear from us. Thank you for your cooperation."

The exec excused me, and I left wondering what else Carolyn might have said about me. Larry was right: I had bet-ter be more careful.

First there were two girls in bathing suits to flirt with, then there were none.

CHAPTER 5

In the Mood

On the Friday morning of that three-day liberty before my little chat with the exec and the public safety officer about the raid at Short Creek, Mom made a late breakfast of scrambled eggs with cheese, hot biscuits and gravy, apricot jam, and milk. Dad had worked the swing shift and I'd had a seven-and-a-half-hour drive the night before, so we both had gone to bed around one a.m. My sisters had gotten up earlier and eaten Kellogg's Frosted Flakes and toast and jam, then returned to their rooms, so it was just the three of us.

I was telling them about Carolyn and Suzy at the pool, and how I'd joked about having three wives at Short Creek. I thought my folks would laugh, but instead they exchanged a meaningful look. What, exactly, that look conveyed, I will never know. We'd never talked about sex, and state-mandated public-school sex education did not exist yet. Locker room talk was a long, and problematic, tradition even back then—my football buddies bragged about screwing half the school, even though we all knew it was a bunch of baloney. (Truth be told, most of us were virgins.) No adult had ever sat me down and explained the birds and the bees, though I'd learned plenty on the farm from watching the cows and the sheep. Anyway, premarital abstinence was the only acceptable choice within the Mormon community.

Mom got up from the table and took the pitcher of milk from the counter to refill my glass. "There is a stake youth dance in Long Beach tonight. You should go. Maybe you'll find a girlfriend and then you'd come home more often."

Dad added, "Why don't you call Ora Beth and ask her to go with you?"

"Dad," I said, rolling my eyes, "you know she's engaged."

"According to her dad, she would take her ring off for you."

"You know me better than that. I wouldn't do that to her or any girl, that's unconscionable! I broke up with her when I moved right after high school. I will not open that wound."

"Fine, then don't ask her," said Mom. "There will be plenty of other girls to dance with."

All's fair in love and war, so I wore my dress blues. There were more girls than boys there, and a few girls even asked me to dance. I was having a great time when I noticed one girl, in particular. She stood out from the rest. She wore a simple yet stylish skirt and blouse, and she had short dark hair and the kind of natural, fresh-faced prettiness that implies good health. She was sitting with a boy I knew from Compton High, and I wondered if she was Scott's date or if they were just friends. I walked over and said hello, glancing down at her left hand—no ring.

"You mind if I ask her to dance?" I said to Scott.

"Ask her, not me," he replied.

I offered my hand. "Hi, my name's Herb. Care to dance?"

"Hi, Herb. I'd like that," she said. "I'm Joyce."

Just as we headed to the dance floor, her hand in mine,

the band began playing the first few notes of "In the Mood." It's one of those songs you can't help but snap your fingers to, the perfect instrumental for dancing the Lindy Hop, which we called the jitterbug. I gently pulled her toward me, and she took my other hand, her expression full of joy. We danced as if we had been dancing together forever, our feet fast, her skirt swirling around her legs as she spun around and around.

From that first spin, I knew I wanted to see her again. Near the end of the song, I leaned toward her and, to be heard over the music, said loudly, "Would you go out with me tomorrow?"

Well, I'd forgotten that, near the end of "In the Mood," the music gets soft, then pauses for a couple of seconds, almost as though Glenn Miller knew we'd need a moment to catch our breaths. Then the band starts playing loud again. I just so happened to put my heart on my sleeve right as the music dropped to nothing, and everyone in the room heard me ask her out.

She just laughed.

When the song ended, for real this time, I walked her back to Scott. "You guys looked great out there," he said. "I can't do the jitterbug, so when the music is fast, you two should dance together."

That was what I wanted to hear.

A few songs later, the band started playing "Tenderly," one of the most romantic songs of all time. My eyes turned to Joyce; her eyes followed me as I approached. I offered her my hand.

We walked out onto the dance floor, and she stepped close to me as the tenor saxophone began to play in perfect harmony with the piano. I held her and we danced as though alone, cheek to cheek, her hand around the back of my neck, my hand gently but firmly on her lower back. I felt overcome, mesmerized by the low, sultry notes of the sax; the scent of her shampoo; the warmth of her closeness. That dance told us all we needed to know.

Looking back, I have three questions: First, why would they play such a sensuous song at a church dance? The bishop himself was playing the saxophone! Second, why didn't a chaperon separate our full-body embrace? Usually a responsible adult would be keeping an eye on things, going around and sticking their hand between too-close couples, saying, *You got to make room for the Holy Ghost.* Third, if Scott liked her, why did he encourage us to dance together?

WHIRLWIND ROMANCE

Joyce and I spent Saturday afternoon at the Pike, the amusement park in Long Beach, and in the evening, we walked on the beach and Rainbow Pier, a three-quarter-mile-long half-circle that extends a quarter mile into the Pacific. She tucked her arm in mine as we strolled along, watching the red sun meet the blue-black water on the horizon. As the twilight faded into darkness, we turned around to take in the city lights, all while getting to know each other.

I had set an age limit for who was appropriate to date at seventeen, which, by today's standards, is considered very young but back then and within the Mormon community was marriageable. I was only nineteen, after all. I liked Joyce enough to rankle at my own self-imposed mandate, however, so instead of asking her age, I asked her if she had graduated this year. Anyway, I justified to myself, there are three questions you never ask a woman: *How much do you weigh? How old are you?* and *Are you pregnant?*

"I'll be a senior this fall," she answered.

"Oh," I said, oh so casually. "When's your birthday?"

"Columbus Day, the twelfth of October."

I conveniently assumed that she was seventeen going on eighteen. That is, until a month later when I'd made the seven-hour drive to ostensibly visit my parents but really to see Joyce. I was standing in her mother's kitchen, sipping a glass of 7UP while Joyce finished getting ready.

"Things are going awfully fast," Larraine said, hands on hips and gaze locked on mine. "You know that my daughter is only sixteen, right?"

I nearly choked on an ice cube. "I . . . I thought she was seventeen."

"She will be seventeen on October the twelfth, and that's too young for how serious you two are getting. She *will* graduate from high school, understand?"

As time passed, Larraine and I did bond somewhat. She resigned herself to the fact that she was going to have me for a son-in-law, then seemed to get excited about it. Her husband worked long hours, leaving her to tend the two younger kids, and her teenage daughter wasn't all that interested in chatting with Mom, so she came to rely on me for adult conversations. Soon she was paying more attention to me, which I think Joyce preferred—that meant that Larraine wasn't paying attention to, and criticizing, her.

I had three days of liberty every other week, and for five months, between visits, Joyce and I wrote each other love letters. First-class mail cost six cents and took one day to travel between Goodyear, Arizona, and Compton, California, plenty of time to build anticipation and for me to miss her. I soon decided that I was ready to take things to the next level, which I did via the postal service, spelling out my question two letters at a time on the back flap of the envelopes. Later, Joyce told me that the mailman, when handing her a letter with "U" and "M" on the envelope, asked, "Are you going to say yes?"

"Say yes to what?"

"Well, um," he said, suddenly nervous, like maybe he was wishing he hadn't stuck his nose in her business. "So far the

envelopes have had 'W,' 'I,' 'L,' 'L' and 'U' and 'M' . . . Could the
next word be anything but 'marry'?"

I'd timed it so I could get my answer Thanksgiving
weekend.

Two weeks before Christmas—Joyce was now officially
seventeen, and I had just turned twenty—she and I were walking down Ocean Boulevard to the Roxy movie theater, hand in
hand. The night was warm but breezy, with the smell of the sea
lingering in the air. Joyce was wearing a light cardigan over her
dress, the sky-blue shade bringing out the blue of her eyes. We
were deliriously happy.

Right before the theater, we passed a jewelry store, and
Joyce stopped at the window. "Look, Herb," she said, pointing
to the engagement rings on display. "You know, Christmas is
just around the corner . . ."

It didn't take a genius to understand what she was saying.
"Which one is your favorite?" I asked. She looked thoughtful
as she assessed the jewelry. I checked my watch. "We have time
before the movie, if you want to go inside?" I said. She smiled.

After the movie, we drove out to La Mirada, where dirt
roads around a square mile of citrus orchards would give us
some privacy. (For any great-grandchildren who might be reading this: in my day, we called what people did at night alone in
cars "necking.") I had just shut off the engine and taken a single
deep inhale of the grapefruit-scented breeze when a car pulled
up behind us. I thought they were another couple until two
men in dark suits got out, the sound of their doors slamming
loud in the evening's quiet. I looked around—we were alone,
as intended, and I didn't see anything that could be used as
a weapon. By the time I'd located a flashlight under the front
seat, one of the men was tapping on my window with his left
hand, holding an FBI badge up to the glass with his right. I
rolled down my window just enough so we could talk.

"What can I do for you, Officer?" I said.

"We're here to ask you some questions related to security clearance."

"This is an odd time and place to be asking me questions." He was probably not used to back talk and gave me a stern look. "But here you are," I conceded.

"Please step out of the car, sir," he said. There, underneath twenty-five-foot-tall grapefruit trees, the two men asked mostly about if and when Joyce and I were planning on getting married. "Did you follow us to the jewelry store today?" I asked but did not receive a reply. When they found out I'd put a down payment on three rings—an engagement ring and two wedding bands—they moved on to asking about what kinds of activities my soon-to-be in-laws were involved in.

"To your knowledge," the second FBI agent asked Joyce, "have your parents ever attended any meetings or social events with known Communist Party members?" Joyce looked at me, bewildered. This was six years after President Truman issued the Loyalty Order that mandated vetting of all federal employees' loyalty to the government, and the height of the Red Scare, when any whiff of Communist ties was grounds for rejection, dismissal, or worse. The Soviet Union, our ally in World War II, was now our enemy, with its own nuclear arsenal. As the United States Army fought Communist-supported forces abroad, the House Un-American Activities Committee, led by Senator Joseph R. McCarthy, rooted out suspected Communists, many of whom worked as intellectuals or creatives. Julius and Ethel Rosenberg had been found guilty of espionage and executed at Sing Sing around the time Joyce and I first met.

Little more than a week after my surprise visit from the FBI, my chief told me, "Just got the notice that you passed security clearance. You are going to be transferred in mid-January to anti-submarine warfare training at Memphis Naval Air Station. The training is fourteen weeks long."

"Do you know where I'll be stationed afterward?" I asked, hoping it would be close to Joyce.

"That depends on where you're needed."

Looking back and tracing the data, Joyce's mother's concern was justified. Joyce and I spent less than thirty days together in person, between our first meeting at the summer dance and Christmas, when we got engaged. Still, Joyce's father, Herald, and Larraine seemed unperturbed when Joyce opened her present on Christmas Day. That afternoon, she drove over to my folks' house to model her shiny new solitaire yellow-gold engagement ring for my parents.

SCHOOL DAYS

I took a week of leave before heading to Memphis. Having been stationed there before, I had no trouble getting there and checking in. There were only five students in the class. Because I was now engaged, dating and USO dances were off my agenda, and I rarely left the base. There was no TV in the barracks, but I could see a movie for ten cents; movies changed three times a week, so I saw a lot of movies. I used the woodworking shop that was open to enlisted personnel to make picture frames and jewelry boxes for Joyce and Mom.

There was also homework. The fourteen weeks went by fast.

I soon found out why the navy had sicked the FBI on me. The sonobuoys and torpedoes we studied weren't a secret in and of themselves; it was the devices' particulars of speed, depth, distance, frequencies, and so on. A sonobuoy is a small buoy five inches in diameter and three feet long. Upon impact with the water after being dropped from an aircraft, it will deploy the electronic sensor and transmitter inside it. The electronic sensor will drop a determined depth in the water and the transmitter will float above, the two parts attached by a fine cable. The sensor can detect and identify a submarine and its location, and track its movement, sending the data as it is collected to the aircraft via the transmitter. Once the submarine is located, the torpedo, equipped with a pattern of sound detectors on its nose, is deployed. It detects sounds coming from the submarine or uses sonar to locate and determine its movements. Once it has homed in, it will track the target and destroy it.

Obviously, the navy didn't want information about how this technology functioned to get into the wrong hands. Even so, I was perplexed to find, about a month after taking the class, an advertisement on the back of *Life* magazine for the torpedo manufacturer showing an image of the torpedo and, roughly, describing how it worked. The first thing I thought was *My date and I were interrupted so I could get clearance to study this torpedo, and now it's on the back of* Life *magazine?*

About a week before the class ended, the five of us received our new assignments. I was assigned to FAETUPAC, Fleet Airborne Electronics Training Unit (Pacific), at Naval Air Station Whidbey Island, in Oak Harbor, Washington. Home of six squadrons of Lockheed P2V Neptune maritime patrol and anti-submarine warfare aircraft, FAETUPAC was responsible for training the crews and certifying instrument flying.

I was able to tack on an extra week of leave to the ten days I had to transfer to the Whidbey Island naval base. The weekends that bookended my leave would be spent in transit, and I hoped to visit Joyce during the two weeks in between. I had left my car with my folks when I was in Memphis, so now I had my car back and, with it, the freedom to go where I wanted, when I wanted, with whomever I wanted. But with her schedule of school by day and homework by night—her mother's words "She *will* graduate from high school, understand?" echoed in my head—we didn't get to see each other all that much. Joyce and I really only had one weekend together.

Mom and Dad were pleased as punch. Dad worked nights, and so, while my sisters were in school, I hung out with my parents, mostly playing pinochle, my mom's favorite. I took them to visit a couple navy ships that were anchored in Long Beach. The first was a destroyer tender called the USS *Bryce Canyon*, and on the way out, my mother tried to convince a drunk first-class boatswain mate that the ship was named after my dad's great-grandfather. I don't think he bought her story, but that didn't stop him from flirting outrageously with her while my dad looked on, laughing. After a tour of an aircraft carrier, my folks took me to Knott's Berry Farm for boysenberry pie à la mode.

The two and a half weeks flew by, and soon enough, I was saying my goodbyes to my family, throwing my seabag in the trunk, setting the bag of snacks Mom put together on the back seat, and heading over to Joyce's to pick her up and take her to school. We'd arranged to get there an hour early so we would have time to do our goodbyes in private. We had settled on September 4 for our wedding.

It would be three and a half months before we would see each other again.

The Federal-Aid Highway Act had not yet passed, so there were no freeways, and I had no idea how long the drive would take. I'd read about the world's tallest trees and decided to take a detour through the Redwood National Park. Not only did I drive through the park, I drove through a redwood tree, its trunk so large that the road had been laid straight through it.

When I stopped at a Standard service station in Crescent City to fill up my gas tank, I picked up a free road map of Oregon. The 1985 movie *Back to the Future* got the service station scene right. "Service" was in the name for a reason. Not only did the attendant fill my gas tank, he checked my radiator, oil, fan belt, tire pressure, then washed all my windows, then showed me how to get on Highway 101. As he folded up the map, he told me, "When you stop again to fill your tank, pick up a Washington map."

"Thanks," I said, excited to get back on the road. I'd spent most of my young life in the deserts of Arizona and California, and I was looking forward to living on an island way up north. I'd never even been north of San Francisco! I headed to Grants Pass to pick up Highway 99, driving up through Eugene to Portland, passing Mount St. Helens (which still had its top), then up through Olympia and Tacoma and Seattle and beyond, stopping every now and then to stretch my legs and take in the sights. My sense of awe only grew as I passed trees three hundred feet tall and so thick that their limbs overlapped. There was water everywhere, rivers and streams running and rain falling blue or brown or gray, depending on the light. The air smelled not like sunshine and dust but like damp, like soil. The evergreens were a deep winter green; the moss that grew on weathered wooden buildings was a nuclear green. Even the cracks in the sidewalk were green.

In Mukilteo, a small town twenty-five miles north of Seattle, I boarded a ferry for my first-ever ferry ride. I had already fallen in love with the Pacific Northwest.

CHAPTER 6

Marriage and Beyond

The date was set for September 4, 1954. In part, this was a pragmatic decision. Joyce's dad, Herald, closed his auto shop for only four holidays: Thanksgiving, Christmas, Fourth of July, and Labor Day. In 1954, Labor Day was on September 6, so that Saturday would be ideal in terms of it being part of a long weekend. But it was more than that. Larraine and Herald had a three-year-old adoptive daughter whom they wanted to seal to them in Mormon tradition so that she would spend her afterlife with them in the celestial kingdom where God dwells "for all time and eternity." They could marry off their eldest and seal their youngest in a single weekend, thereby killing two birds with one stone.

In the meantime, I'd fulfill my assignment and write to Joyce. I didn't have a lot to say—navy life on the home front wasn't all that exciting, as I'd hoped—so I bought cards down at the ship store and scribbled out short little notes, just to let her know I was thinking of her.

There were no Link Trainers at the Naval Air Station Whidbey Island. I had to learn how to operate another machine, this time a flight trainer for pilots, navigators, and radar operators. Remember, this was 1954—we were using vacuum tubes, not transistors (computer chips) in our electronics; turntables and vinyl records, not tape or digital sound. The flight trainer was operated by a huge bank of electronics that, the TD2 petty officer claimed, had over one hundred vacuum tubes. I believed it, though I had more to do than count them. The sounds needed for anti-submarine lessons were on sixteen-inch vinyl records, played on professional turntables and using the highest quality headphones available.

Soon after moving into the barracks, an old salt by the name of Alex saw me emptying my pockets and dropping the change into a two-gallon jar in my locker. He stopped and asked, "Couldn't find a piggy bank big enough?"

"Nah! Gotta save a lotta coins by September for my honeymoon. You know, my salary would only get us a couple nights at a cheap hotel. I only have three and a half months, hope I make it."

"Bryce, outta my way." Alex dug into his pocket, then dropped a few coins in the jar. "That'll get you a little bit closer."

Later that afternoon, Alex brought four other guys by my bed. "Bryce, I told these fellas about your 'piggy bank.' Open your locker and show them." They watched with interest as I turned the dial and swung the locker door open to reveal the jar with an inch or so of change at the bottom. "OK, you guys," Alex said, "your change goes in the piggy bank. We gotta give enough for at least a good bottle of champagne."

By taps the next night, there was a good handful of coins on my bed. More coins appeared as word traveled through the barracks until I was getting between three and five dollars a night. A couple guys taped a picture of a pink piggy bank to the jar to make it official. By September, it held over $400, more than four months of my navy salary. I'd be able to buy that good bottle of champagne and then some.

WHEW, WE PULLED IT OFF

September arrived in the blink of an eye. Two and a half weeks of leave were granted. Rings purchased. I'd written to my bride-to-be to find out if I could get my blood test done by the navy and bring the results with me. Her answer was yes. That would give us three or four more days for our honeymoon. All we needed was the license and we would be ready for the wedding.

Talk about naïve. The day before our wedding, we went to the Civic Center, the tallest building in Los Angeles, to get our marriage license. We arrived long before the doors opened, thinking that we would wait hand in hand in the early-morning sunshine, then be the first couple inside, able to quickly check this errand off our to-do list. Then we'd have the whole day ahead of us to manage any last-minute details, no sweat.

Of course, our mothers had to come with us because of our ages. Joyce would not be eighteen for another month, and I would be twenty-one in November. Perhaps this should've slowed us down—as I tell young folks, if you have to get a parent's signature to get married, then you are too damn young to get married. We also didn't factor in the fact that LA County was the most populated area in the state, and the line was already long, made up of grumpy people rubbing their eyes and yawning. Then, when we finally made it inside, the clerk rejected my blood test report from the navy.

"I can't accept this," she said. "You have to get a physician to sign the application at least three days before your wedding." Panic ensued.

"But—" I said.

"I thought—" said Joyce.

"What do—" said my mother.

"That can't—" said Joyce's mom.

"QUIET!" the clerk shouted.

I held up my hand so we wouldn't all talk over one another again. "Our wedding is tomorrow," I said.

The clerk looked less than impressed. "You can get the blood test waived," she said, reaching under the counter and pulling out a couple sheets of paper, which she slid across to me. "You just need a magistrate to sign the waiver."

"Thank you," I said, but she'd already shifted her attention elsewhere. "Next!" she called as the four of us turned toward the exit.

In another room full of waiting people, an assistant with a clipboard approached us and asked how she could help. After we told her our problem, she turned a few pages, slid her finger down the page, and said, "I can squeeze you in Tuesday afternoon." Pandemonium broke out again.

I motioned for everyone to calm down. "We can't solve the problem by yelling," I said. "Tomorrow we'll just have to have a mock wedding and reception, and not tell a soul. Joyce and I can get married next week."

Larraine and my mom did not think this was a good plan. While we were discussing it, a man in a suit and tie and carrying a briefcase walked past us and out the door. "Is that a magistrate?" I asked the assistant.

"Yes, but—"

I took off after him. He was already all the way at the other end of the hallway, waiting for the elevator. The doors opened with a ping. He waited patiently as the passengers exited, then stepped inside. The doors began to close . . .

The soles of my shoes squeaked on the marble floor as I slid the last few feet and stuck my hand between the doors. They opened with a sigh, and I entered the elevator and took a deep breath to collect myself. The magistrate eyed me warily. "Sir," I began with a nod, calling on my navy-trained manners. "I'm sorry to bother you, but I am on a brief leave from the navy so that I can get married." He nodded for me to continue, and I told him my story on the way down to the lobby. "Let me see the navy blood test report," he said. I handed it to him, and he glanced over it. "This is irrational." He looked at me. "This proves that you met the requirement."

"Yes, sir."

"Hand me the waiver and turn around." I did as instructed, and the magistrate used my back as a writing surface to sign the paper.

"Thank you very much, sir," I said.

"Thank you for serving our country," he replied, handing me the signed form. "Have a wonderful wedding, and give my regards to the bride."

In the lobby stood Joyce and our mothers. "You got him to sign it," Mom blurted out.

"What makes you think so?"

"You're smiling ear to ear and your face is lit up like a neon sign."

"Yes! We are going to have a real wedding tomorrow!"

We got married the next day, in the cultural hall of the chapel in Compton. It was a simple Mormon ceremony, not the kind you see today where people pick and choose what to include and write their own vows. Forty people or so were in attendance, and Scott, the guy who'd been at the dance with Joyce when we first met, was my best man. My sister Patsy was Joyce's maid of honor. A couple new friends from the navy came—one of them fell asleep in his seat in the back. After we said our I do's, we had a good old-fashioned Mormon reception, organized by the women's Relief Society, with hors d'oeuvres and 7Up with lime sherbet cut into squares bobbing around the bowl—there might not have been any alcohol, but

there was plenty of sugar. The next day, a Sunday, we went
to church, and on Monday, we drove eight hours to Mesa,
Arizona, for the sealing, the Mormon ritual of joining people
(and their progeny) for all of eternity.

Most weddings have a glitch that you laugh about later
in life. Other than the fuss with the blood test, the wedding
was perfect. Well, except for one gift: a small black-and-white
puppy from my sister Phyllis.

HOME SWEET HOME

We spent the week of our honeymoon in the family's cabin
in the San Jacinto Mountains just west of Palm Springs, then
took our time on the drive from Southern California to the
Pacific Northwest, camping out for three nights along the
way. We'd picked up our new puppy from my parents' house,
and quickly realized that traveling with an un-house-trained
puppy was very trying. The back seat was full of Joyce's stuff,
so Snoopy was either on her lap or on a towel on the front
floorboard. The puppy used the towel more than once, after
which we'd stop at a service station or a creek so that I could
wash it, then hang it over the back window and roll the window up real tight so we wouldn't lose it, air-drying it as we
drove. When the outside half was dry, we would flip the towel
to air-dry the other end.

I'd prepped our new house trailer the week before our
wedding. Because of the Korean War, the personnel on the
base had almost doubled, which caused a big increase in the
need for married housing, so the navy had purchased a large
quantity of twenty-eight-foot one-bedroom house trailers
and set them up on the east side of the island, at the seaplane
base, near the emergency hospital and main sick bay and the
navy exchange, and within walking distance to the town of

Oak Harbor. Ault Field, where I worked, was to the north-west side of the island, near Deception Pass State Park and the Deception Pass Bridge, which crossed over to Fidalgo Island. After a couple of weeks in the trailer, I was awakened in the middle of the night by some strange noises. I got up to see what was going on, leaving the light off and closing the bedroom door behind me so as not to disturb Joyce—that was mistake number one—and headed down the hall to turn on the bathroom light—that was mistake number two. On my second step, my right foot landed in something squishy; I felt it oozing between my toes, a sensation that had my stomach lurching just as the scent of dog doo reached my nose. Hopping on my left foot, I made it to the bathroom, where I turned on the bathroom light. *Oh my God!* Shredded toilet paper and sanitary napkins littered the floor. Snoopy must have smelled blood and traced it to its source in the trash can, then proceeded to rip them apart and scatter them around the room.

First things first: I wrapped my right foot in a bathroom towel so I wouldn't spread puppy poop all over the floor. Snoopy was blissfully unaware of his wrongdoing, and he was still shaking a napkin in his jaws as though it were a rabbit whose neck he was trying to break. I caught him, then hopped toward the door, puppy in my left hand, my right hand holding the towel around my foot. Mistake number three: I put Snoop outside so I could clean up the mess and take a shower.

By now, Joyce was awake and standing in the bedroom doorway. "Go on back to bed, Joyce," I said. "I'm taking care of it." After getting everything including me cleaned up, I went outside to retrieve Snoopy, but he was nowhere to be found. Rather than standing outside in the middle of the night in a navy trailer park yelling "Snooooopy!" at the top of my lungs, I figured that by morning he would come home. We never saw Snoopy again.

HAPPY NEWS

About a month after my birthday, Joyce threw up. On the third day of her vomiting, we headed to urgent care. This was Joyce's first visit to the base's medical bay, so she filled out the forms while I waited. In the examination room, the doctor flipped through the paperwork and took Joyce's vitals. He made a note, then raised his head and, with a big smile, asked, "When was your last period?"

Joyce thought for a while. "Sometime around Halloween," she replied.

"Your wedding band looks new," the doctor said, looking at me. "How long have you been married?"

"Three months. Why?"

"Well, I suspect that you are pregnant. We'll take a test to be sure."

"How long before we know?"

"We'll have the test results before noon tomorrow. I'm sure you're pregnant, but wait until we get the positive results before you buy any diapers." I squeezed Joyce's hand, and she beamed. The doctor added, "The way your faces lit up, I'm guessing congratulations are in order?"

"Yes, thank you," Joyce said. "Thank you!"

"Don't thank me, thank your husband. Stop at the nurses' desk and they will set up your prenatal appointment schedule. That way, if the results are positive, they'll have your schedule ready."

On the way home, we talked all about having a baby. As I left for work the next day, Joyce was in the bathroom throwing up. When I returned that afternoon, she met me at the door, jumping up and down and waving her prenatal schedule. "I tested positive; we're going to have a baby!" She already had a list of names, be it a girl or boy. I don't need to tell you what the conversation was about that evening.

Joyce's morning sickness was over with, at least the throwing-up part, by mid-April. Which was great because we could pick up where we left off exploring the Pacific Northwest. Our first trip was to Butchart Gardens, on Vancouver Island, Canada. Joyce said she felt like she had died and gone to heaven. The North Cascades Highway opened the first week of May, and we packed the wicker picnic basket that Snoopy had come in (yes, I washed it) with a picnic and spent the night in Winthrop. We drove up through Deception Pass Park and took the Anacortes ferry to Friday Harbor on San Juan Island for lunch, which made us feel like big spenders.

Joyce was an animal person. Having a pet helped her cope with being home alone while I was at work and on duty every fourth night. Instead of a puppy, she chose to get a cat, who turned out to be another wrecking ball. She loved to run to the couch, jump with all her claws extended, and use the backrest as a springboard. The furniture she was quickly destroying belonged to the navy, and the veterinarian in Mount Vernon would not trim her claws but did say he could find a farmer who would be happy to adopt her. "She sounds like she'd be a good mouser," he said.

Joyce agreed—the cat seemed less interested in cuddling than in pouncing and clawing. "What about a kitten?" she asked the vet.

"I don't know of any kittens being given away at the moment," he said, then paused. "However . . . if you're interested, a man just brought in a litter of baby skunks to have their scent glands removed. Skunks make great pets; they love to be petted and to sit in your lap. You must keep them indoors, though, because if they wander off, they usually don't come home, and without scent glands, they have no protection from predators. They should be ready for adoption early next week."

"Can we talk it over and call you back tomorrow?"

"Sure, but I want to warn you: however cuddly they may be, owning a skunk is not like owning a dog or cat."

Joyce picked out her favorite female and christened her Penelope. She fit in the palm of my hand. We prepaid for neutering and vaccinations so we would be sure to come back in a few months, then left with our new skunk, a bag of litter, a small pet bed, a couple of pet toys, and a pink collar and leash.

With a baby on the way, we knew that we'd need to rent a bigger place. Nothing was available on base, but we were put on the waiting list. We did find an ad for a small one-bedroom guesthouse on a farm, about eight miles from base. After a visit, we decided to move in. Our new rental was perched on a cliff overlooking Penn Cove and, to the south, the small town of Coupeville. The owners, the Zelstras, were plowing a plot of land between our place and the edge of the cliff and asked if we would like to plant a spring garden. Joyce, who had that second-trimester energy, dug right in. Penelope loved the fresh vegetables, especially the green peas. I learned that my wife had a green thumb—and that sometimes there can be too much of a good thing. What are you supposed to do with twenty heads of lettuce and two dozen zucchinis?

AND THEN THERE WERE THREE

In the middle of the night of August 12, Joyce shook me awake. "I think I'm in labor!" she said excitedly.

I sat up, my heart racing. "Should we head for the hospital?"

"It's OK, Herb." She patted my arm. "The contractions aren't close enough together yet. The doctor said five minutes apart, lasting for one minute, for one hour or longer."

By the time we got to the entrance gate at the seaplane base, where the hospital was, Joyce's contractions were one minute apart. The marine guard refused to let us in because the rules state that no nonmilitary women were allowed on base before 08:00, unless it was an emergency. I tried talking sense into him while Joyce gasped and moaned. Quickly I realized his head was just too hard for reason.

"My wife's in labor, you idiot!" I shouted.

"Rules are rules," he shouted back. "It has to be an emergency!"

"This *is* an emergency, can't you see that?"

Our argument got so loud that the sergeant came out and asked what the ruckus was all about. Without thinking, I said, "My wife is having contractions one minute apart, and this stupid idiot won't let us in! Either we get to the hospital, or the baby is going to be born right here, and I hope to hell that one of you knows how to deliver a baby because I sure don't!"

The sergeant looked old and tired enough to have kids himself. "Contractions five minutes or less apart is an emergency," he told the young, overeager guard. "Get her to the hospital, GO!"

I loved the sound of the sergeant giving the guard hell as we drove off.

At the emergency room, the nurse took one look at Joyce and grabbed a wheelchair. "Go wait in the maternity waiting room," she called to me over her shoulder as she wheeled my wife toward the delivery room. Before I could even get to the waiting room, another nurse stopped me. "Your wife just gave birth to a baby girl. Seven pounds, nine and a half ounces."

"A baby girl!"

"That's right," the nurse said with a smile. "After we get your daughter cleaned up, you can come down to the nursery and view her. She'll join your wife in her room once she's recovered, and you can visit them there." Vicki was born at 07:53, forty weeks after my birthday. My birthday wish had come true.

BABY BLUES

Joyce and Vicki stayed in the hospital for three days, leaving with a seven-dollar medical bill. A few days after coming home, I checked on the baby and discovered that, somehow, Penelope had gotten in the crib. This, of course, was a major concern. We were aware of the danger of cats around babies, but we'd never heard of the danger of skunks around babies. The veterinarian in Mount Vernon gladly took Penelope back. She was our last pet until I graduated from college.

Our little guesthouse had a beautiful view of the cove and fir trees surrounding the property, but Joyce needed more than a beautiful view. It was hard on her, an eighteen-year-old alone with a newborn and no neighbors to call and few friends. Of the two couples we got to know, both wives worked. On top of that, we only had one car, so if Joyce wanted to leave the property during the day, she had to drop me off at the base and pick me up. Every fourth day, I was gone for two whole days and a night. When I was home, I tried to help as much as I could, picking Vicki up in the night and changing her diaper before bringing her to Joyce to nurse. Even so, as the days passed, Joyce seemed to get more and more overwhelmed, more exhausted, more taciturn. Sometimes I'd get home to find her still in her nightgown, her hair unwashed, the dishes piled high in the sink.

In the 1950s, the "baby blues," or postpartum depression, wasn't talked about, even at postnatal checkups. In fact, the psychiatric community did not officially recognize postpartum depression until 1994. There weren't yet any medications for depression, and religious leaders looked at it as a weakness or caused by evil spirits. I had no idea what was happening to my wife, and no experience with depression myself, and no way to help her as much as I wanted to. She was inside of it, alone for long stretches, and without any support. Her mother would have probably scolded or criticized her had Joyce called her—which she didn't bother to do. I wish we'd known better and gotten her the help she and so many new mothers need, but that just wasn't an option at the time. Therefore, we lived with it the best we could.

UP-ANCHOR, DESTINATION COLLEGE

One thing that cheered Joyce up was our outings around Western Washington. Time flew by, and before we knew it, May 5, 1956, was upon us. On May 1, my skipper stopped by my office to try to talk me into reenlisting. After discussing my goals in life and the pro and cons of going to college, I commented, "Lieutenant Selkirk, sir, no disrespect, but if I see you walking down the sidewalk in Oak Harbor next week, I'll say, *Hi, Jim.*"

"Point well taken, Bryce. Hope you graduate summa cum laude. Stop by when you pick up your discharge papers and say goodbye."

Some of the perks of being a petty officer were that you got travel pay to go where you were enlisted, and the navy covered moving costs when you were honorably discharged. We had one week to move out of our apartment. Bright and early on Monday morning, we got a call from Housing that there would be a civil service crew at our apartment on Thursday at 09:00. We were to place anything we wanted to take with us in a corner of the living room and make another pile for everything else.

Right on time, there was a man at our door with a clipboard saying that he needed to survey what we were shipping. "Right there," I said, pointing to the items neatly stacked on the couch. He eyed them, then pointed to the other pile. "Are you sure that's all you don't want packed? Once everything is loaded up, there is no adding or removing." I looked at Joyce, who nodded.

While he was making his list, three other men set up a makeshift shop on the lawn and began unloading two-by-fours and sheets of plywood. After reviewing the list, they started building a huge box. It took them two hours to build a box approximately eight feet long, seven feet wide, and six feet high with one end open. They loaded all of our stuff into the box, fitting everything in so perfectly that I don't think there was room for even one more pillow. Then they nailed on the end to close it. While we were filling out the paperwork, a forklift loaded the box onto the truck. "When do you plan to be at the receiving address?" the foreman asked.

"That's my parents' address," I told him. "We are headed to Arizona first to find a place to live. So, it will be a week or two."

"It will be there, ready for delivery when you get to your parents' house."

We owned a 1950 Nash "upside-down bathtub." It was ugly, but it was the best buy for the money, with good gas mileage, and the front seats folded all the way back to make a six-foot-plus bed that was wide enough for Joyce, me, and nine-month-old Vicki.

We had the car packed and ready to go within an hour after the truck drove off. We wanted to avoid the urban traffic around Seattle and down through Tacoma and Olympia in the morning, so we left at four p.m. (not 16:00; we were on civilian time now). It was misty and a cool sixty-four degrees. We spent the night just south of Tumwater, waking up before six a.m. to start our fifteen-hundred-mile trip to Tempe, Arizona, finishing off the sandwiches we had packed for breakfast. Vicki had her own supply of snacks and food in Tupperware containers. Food that needed to be kept cool was stored in our secondhand Coleman galvanized cooler. (The Coleman plastic cooler wasn't available until 1957.)

We spent the night just outside of Virginia City, Nevada. When we woke at sunrise, there was a white dusting of snow. We arrived in Tempe that evening and found a motel to use as home base while checking out Arizona State College at Tempe and looking for a place to live.

The next day, we started our search without much luck, the temperature rising by the hour. Our car did not have air-conditioning. We stopped for lunch and to get out of the hundred-degree heat. Joyce pressed her glass of soda, the ice clinking, to her forehead and sighed. Vicki's cheeks were bright red, though she seemed happy enough eating her ham sandwich. "Better get a move on," I said, but just as we got back in the car, it dawned on me that I had helped my football buddy Rae Brimhall's dad, Elias, build a concrete-block rental duplex behind their house when I was stationed at Goodyear. I had been his pro bono hod carrier on my liberty days. "I have an idea," I told Joyce. We parked outside a grocery store so I could use the pay phone and Joyce and Vicki could shop for snacks and cool off.

Maritta, Rae's mother, answered the phone. "Maritta!" I said. "This is a voice from your past, Herb Bryce." After we chatted for a while, I said, "We've looked all over Tempe, and the apartments either don't fit our needs or don't fit our budget. Is there any chance one of the units in the duplex I helped Elias build is available for rent? I'm starting college at ASC this summer."

"Tell you what. Why don't you, Joyce, and Vicki come to dinner tonight? I'm making a King Ranch chicken casserole, there'll be more than enough. I'll talk with Elias when he gets home. After dinner, while our girls take care of Vicki, the four of us can work things out. See you between five thirty and six." She didn't give me a chance to respond before hanging up.

We bought an air conditioner that attached to the car window while we waited for dinner—we were going to need it here in Arizona. During our after-dinner powwow, Elias smiled and said, "Herb, I never did pay you for the work you did on that duplex. How's twenty-five dollars a month for rent, and a promise not to tell anyone?"

"Thank you! Thank you! Thank you! Can we pay you now and move in next week?"

"Give us two days to get it ready. You can move in anytime after that. Your rent starts the fifteenth."

Their daughter Macella added, "I'm available if you need a babysitter."

"Me, too," said her twin, Marita.

I called my aunt and uncle Stella and Grant to see if we could visit and show off Vicki. My real motive was to see if I could borrow Grant's flatbed stake truck, the one we used to move beehives. At their place, Grant checked his calendar and said he wouldn't need it for at least two weeks. "I can use my pickup if anything comes up," he assured me, throwing in a canvas tarp cover and ropes just in case. I had called my father-in-law, Herald, to see if he knew anyone with a forklift we could borrow or rent to load the box onto the truck, and he said he was pretty sure a friend who owned a large construction company had one.

I filled the gas tank and parked it out back by the honey extractor and storage building, then we headed back to the Brimhalls' to see if we could empty our car and store our stuff in the apartment. "Sure," Maritta said. "It's clean. All we need is to get the gas and electric meters read, which is scheduled for tomorrow. Cella and Marita are going to wash the windows tomorrow, too. Then it'll be ready for you."

"Thanks again," I said, noting Vicki's thousand-mile stare. "I think it's time we get the baby to bed. We will see you soon!"

The next morning, we checked out of the motel, had breakfast, and picked up the truck, parking our Nash under a giant pecan tree at Grant and Stella's place. We put Vicki in her car seat, which, at the time, was just a thin canvas bag with two leg holes sewn onto a narrow metal frame and large metal hooks that fit over the back of the seat. Stella fixed us a big lunch and packed us a box of Cheerios, the tried-and-true baby pacifier, and some soft drinks for the road. Grant hung a wet canvas water bag on the headlight. (The water evaporated off the wet bag and kept the water cool inside.)

I glanced in the rearview mirror as we drove away. There was Grant, Stella, and their two boys waving goodbye as we set out for California to get our huge wooden box.

CHAPTER 7

Education, My Passport to the Future

As we turned the corner, there it was: a giant wooden box sitting on my parents' front lawn. We had called ahead before leaving Tempe to let Mom and Dad know we were on our way and that they should be expecting the box. When we pulled into the driveway, Mom came flying out of the house. She had her hand on the truck's passenger door handle before I'd even turned off the ignition. Vicki was her first grandchild, and this was the first time Mom was meeting her. "Howard!" she shouted back toward the house. "Go get the Polaroid camera!"

Mom was so excited that it scared Vicki, and she started crying. It took most of the morning to calm her down enough to let Grandma hold her. Once she did, they were inseparable. This relieved Joyce, who had spent the entire eight-hour car ride, with only one rest stop, taking care of Vicki while I drove.

The next morning, Mom, Joyce, and Vicki stopped by Herald's garage before going to see Larraine. Joyce's parents had visited us on Labor Day, so they had already met their grandbaby, but that was way back when she was only one month old. Now she was nine months.

I stayed at my folks' house to wait for the forklift. At about ten o'clock, a forest-green truck with a forklift on a trailer pulled up in front of the house. "Hi, I'm Jim," said the operator. "Herald said it was a big box, and he wasn't kidding. What's in it?"

"All our furniture and household belongings."

"Why didn't you rent a moving van? Wouldn't it have been easier, and the movers would do all the work?"

I shrugged. "That's the way the navy does it. It works for them by land or sea."

Jim came equipped with sheets of heavy plywood to cover the lawn. By noon, the box was on the truck, tied down and ready to go. Dad threw two crowbars, a nail puller, a claw hammer, and a four-pound hammer behind the truck seat. "Bring them back the next time you come this way," he said.

It was another eight-hour-plus drive to Mesa, so we waited until Friday morning to head to our new home. My mom waved and blew kisses to Vicki as we pulled out of the driveway. I had called ahead for help, and Rae and Denzel said they could be there on our move-in date, on Saturday morning. We spent the night in a motel, then met them in front of the apartment building bright and early. After some back-thumping among us guys, a polite greeting to Joyce, and a "Hello, sweetheart" for the baby, we got to work.

Rae's twin sisters took Vicki to keep her out of our way, and Joyce stood by in the apartment for when she'd need to direct us about where to put everything. I started banging away at the front panel of the box, to no avail. Eventually we called up Rae's dad, Elias, to come out to help. Even with the four of us working together, we had a hell of a time getting the front off the box. Makes sense—the navy movers built the box to survive the roughest seas, and though we thought we were pretty tough guys, we weren't as tough as that. Finally, we got that dang panel off so we could unload the box, and once it was emptied, Elias called dibs. "Put in a window or two and a door," he said, "and it's the perfect work shed."

Now all we had to do was get the box off the truck. Even empty and with the front panel removed, the thing weighed nearly seven hundred pounds. We used pry bars to tip it, slid four-by-fours with blocks underneath to leverage it, then jumped up and down on top of the planks to lift and slide it—and we probably looked like the Marx Brothers while doing it. We were covered in grime and sweat by the time we were done, with more than a few scrapes and splinters to boot.

I had a month before summer classes started, so I helped Elias convert that beast of a box into a work shed. A footing of concrete blocks, two windows, a door, a sloped roof, a bucket of blue-gray paint, and white paint for the trim, and Elias had a real nice shed.

While Joyce got us settled in our place, I worked for Grant on the bee farm. Joyce seemed to like our new situation, especially when Rae's mother took her under her wing, and apparently, Marita and Macella thought God had sent Vicki just for them to play with. What we might now call "social anxiety" had fully taken ahold of my wife, and she wasn't much for initiating friendships or any kind of socializing. So this built-in community really helped.

That summer, I took a couple early-morning classes at Arizona State to get my GI Bill started, arranging my schedule on the bee farm around school. Pretty soon, I realized that the $164 per month I received from the government wouldn't cover my family's costs, especially when Joyce got morning sickness in August and we knew another kid was on the way. I'd lived with my uncle Jearl and aunt Falene at the end of high school, and just those few years earlier, Jearl's GI Bill had paid for not just rent but everything—room and board, textbooks, even a typewriter and other school supplies. Then colleges figured out that more government money could be funneled to them if they required students to live on campus, and they might as well raise tuition while they were at it. Things got complicated, and by the time I came along, the government essentially said, *Here's a check, you figure out how to stretch it.*

Once fall semester started, I would have to take a full class load, meaning I'd need to work late afternoons and nights. I knew this wasn't going to be easy on Joyce, who started showing in early November. Thank goodness Mrs. Brimhall, Macella, and Marita would be around to help out when Joyce needed a break.

NOT ALL CLASSES ARE CREATED EQUAL

My first class on the first day of fall quarter had the biggest impact on me. As my fellow students and I walked into the lecture hall, there were little explosions with small puffs of purple smoke under our feet. That introduction to chemistry class was a blast, both literally and figuratively. Dr. Duane Brown spent the first day talking about how chemistry related to our everyday lives, how it affected the world around us, and he did a couple of demonstrations. You could tell that he really loved connecting with students. He did make one big mistake, however: he told us the name of the compound that we were stepping on. On my first trip to the library, I found the directions for making nitrogen triiodide, and it didn't take long for there to be a few tiny explosions on the steps to the entrance of the science building.

I had pretty much narrowed down my major to one of the physical sciences. I had enjoyed my high school chemistry and physics classes, but my biology teacher was a dud. He made us memorize the twenty-five-plus parts of a grasshopper, which, in my estimation, was not learning biology. Worse still, he had walked up behind a female student and dropped a snake on the back of her neck. She screamed bloody murder—of course—and he laughed and laughed. Not exactly what I'd call role-model behavior.

After chemistry class came physics. While I was very interested in the subject, the professor taught it in abstractions, not as a part of everyday life. My next-semester physics instructor made it obvious that he was a researcher, and teaching was the price he paid to do research. When the starting bell rang, he walked through the side door, turned his back on us without any kind of greeting, and lectured while writing formulas on the blackboard. When the ending bell rang, he simply turned toward the door and walked out. That class was excellent for teaching me what not to do.

Dr. Brown won me over to chemistry as my major. Eventually he became my academic major advisor, mentor, and close friend. We had several things in common: Both of us had been born to LDS parents. We'd both had college football scholarships—Duane had played for BYU; I played for ASC. We were both naval veterans—Duane had served on a submarine; I taught anti-submarine warfare. Most importantly, we both enjoyed doing chemical demonstrations, and we both loved science and teaching. His example was the one I planned to follow.

FROM SAILOR TO DORM MOM

Bonnie arrived on April 11, 1957, at nine p.m. She was seven pounds, twelve ounces. The Brimhalls had been wonderful landlords, babysitters, and friends, but with another mouth to feed and a strenuous course load, I was excited to start my new job for the fall quarter of my sophomore year.

I was to be a dorm mom.

The previous year, I had taken a battery of placement tests to see what I'd forgotten during my time in the navy before I could enroll in classes. I was waiting to see my advisor to go over the results when an older woman sat down next to me. I guessed her to be in her late sixties or early seventies—absolutely ancient! *She's pretty old to be going to college,* I thought. "Are you waiting for the advisor, too?" I asked.

"Heavens, no!" she said. "I'm way too old to go to college. I'm waiting for my appointment with the dean of students."

"Do you work at the college?"

"Something like that. I'm a resident hall director for a men's dormitory."

"A men's dorm?"

"All the dorm directors are retired or widowed women. Well, except at the men's athletic dorm. We're called 'dorm moms.'"

As our conversation continued, I learned that she got a free apartment and utilities, including a phone, plus a salary. "I wish they had a resident hall director position for a married man with children," I said.

"They just might have one. They're opening a temporary dorm for visitors, next to the married student housing. At our last directors meeting, they didn't have a dorm mom yet. I'd check with the dean of students."

I excused myself and walked over to the dean's assistant's desk to make an appointment. "I've got an appointment to-morrow afternoon at two," I told the dorm mom as I returned to my seat.

"Good luck," she said.

I got the job, but the dorm was under construction. Like me, many veterans were using the GI Bill, and there was a se-rious dearth of housing. All that was available at ASC was re-purposed air force barracks from the World War II era—but

I would have believed you if you told me they'd been built during World War I.

Now, as the fall semester began, two long barracks were ready to welcome visitors and temporary students, mostly for visiting athletes, short-term researchers, foreign groups, traveling actors, and so on. I was the manager, concierge, custodian, and housekeeper, all in one. I carried luggage and changed bedding, fixed leaky faucets and recommended restaurants and gave directions. I would get the same deal as the other dorm moms: free rent, utilities including a phone, and a salary.

It was an ideal job, but the downside was we had to move. My family's housing was an apartment across from the dorm in a married student housing building, where the Grady Gammage Memorial Auditorium, designed by Frank Lloyd Wright, now stands. Not only was Brimhall's apartment much better than the apartment we were moving into, we had developed close ties with the Brimhalls. But free rent and utilities and a salary wasn't something we could pass up.

CHEMISTRY ON REAL LIFE

The one-bedroom apartment needed a whole lot of tender loving care, and we did what we could on our very limited budget. We painted the interior and added wainscoting and wallpapered the kitchen. The kitchen's top cupboards didn't have doors, so we made curtains for them. The old linoleum floor noticeably sloped toward the wall in the eating area, where there was a quarter-inch gap—shine a flashlight on it and you could see the ground below—and we had to put four five-inch-long, quarter-inch-thick steel bars on the stove's four burners to keep pots and pans level. (We didn't need them for baking a two-layer cake; we'd simply rotate the layers so the cake would come out even.) But it was free rent.

We requested maintenance to level the floor and install footing blocks, but they surely had a long to-do list and were slow getting around to our place. Which turned out to be to our benefit.

A group of neighbors invited us to a party, and we volunteered to make homemade root beer. The recipe was very simple: just water, sugar, root beer extract, and yeast. The yeast reacts with the sugar to produce carbon dioxide (CO_2) and ethyl alcohol. The alcohol is less than 2 percent.

We made four gallons, so we bought sixteen thirty-two-ounce glass bottles from the local tavern. (Plastic bottles wouldn't be invented until 1970.) We filled the bottles and sealed them with metal caps, then stored them on top of our kitchen cupboard to ferment. "Five days should do it," I told Joyce, feeling confident. I was a chemistry major, after all.

The temperature outside was a hundred degrees, and our evaporative cooler dropped the temperature only fifteen or twenty degrees. I should have realized that heat rises, and the warmer it is, the faster the mixture ferments, and that CO_2 production builds pressure inside the bottles—and that we'd placed the root beer in the warmest spot in the house. Right after midnight on the fifth day, we were woken by the sound of exploding glass. I jumped out of bed and raced toward the sound. In the kitchen, root beer was soaking into the cupboard curtains and running across the countertops and trickling onto the kitchen floor, heading toward the gap underneath the wall. Shards of glass were everywhere, including stuck in the Celotex ceiling.

The first thing we did was rescue the remaining eleven unbroken bottles and put them in our galvanized tub in the shower, then fill the tub with cold water to bring the temperature down. We washed the root beer off the floor, and I brought in the garden hose to spray the gap under the wall.

Then I headed to a truck-stop service station to buy ice, which we packed around the bottles to stop the fermentation. Once the crisis was under control, I compared the glass shards to the intact bottles—the ones that had broken were made of thinner glass. Good to know for next time.

That afternoon, homemade root beer floats with homemade ice cream were the hit of the party. Two weeks later, maintenance jacked up the floor and put in footing blocks. No more emergency drain.

RODBUSTER (RODMAN) SUMMER 1958

Besides being a dorm mom, I did just about everything to make money. I didn't get to see my family much, or at least not in terms of quality time—I was pretty much always working, going to school, or studying, and when I wasn't, I was sleeping. I worked as a school custodian, discount store go-to guy (from sales to carpenter and everything in between), pizza chef, Caterpillar plow driver for a cotton farmer, and bee farmer. I played semipro football in the American Football League, taking home a portion of the gate; the manager would hand out fifties or a couple twenties as we left the locker room after the game. My favorite role, however, was rodbuster.

A couple of weeks before the end of the spring semester of my junior year, I'd finished cultivating more than a thousand acres, getting the fields ready to plant cotton, and now I needed to cram for finals. By the time class let out, I was ready for a break, and Joyce and I decided to take a week off to visit our families in Compton. It had been nine months since our folks had seen the girls. The grandparents were excited to see and hold their two granddaughters. Vicki was almost three, and Bonnie was just over a year.

Tuesday evening, Herald asked me at dinner if I'd be interested in staying through the summer. "You could earn some good money," he said.

The first thing I thought was *He's going to offer me a job in his auto shop.* Though I was quick to learn handywork, I was far from being a car mechanic, and I wasn't too sure being Herald's employee would do our relationship any favors, so I hedged. "That depends on the job," I said.

"You remember Jim?"

"Yeah, the guy who brought the forklift to load the box on the truck when we were moving."

"Right. Well, he came into the shop this morning because his truck wasn't running on all six cylinders. We got to talking about that big box and how you jumped right in to get it secured on the truck. I guess you impressed him, and he's looking for a rodbuster to work on a skyscraper in Los Angeles this summer."

"What's a rodbuster?"

"Someone who ties reinforcement steel bars."

"Oh, tying rebar. Sure, I could do that. I've worked mostly with wire mesh for floors and driveways, though we did use rebars for foundations and footings when Dad had his concrete business. Did Jim say what the pay is?"

"An apprentice salary. That's two dollars and sixty-eight cents an hour."

I put down my fork and wiped my mouth with my napkin. The new dorms were finished, and so my dorm mom job had ended, and I was seeking another gig. Joyce was looking at me, her eyebrows raised. We were both doing the math: one week's salary would pay for four months' rent for our married-student housing. Living with family meant free room and board for the summer. My parents owned a two-bedroom house, and Joyce's parents owned a three-bedroom house, making theirs the better option. Which meant, for better or worse, living with

Joyce's parents. They didn't have the best of relationships, but Joyce could take the kids to the beach or the San Diego Zoo or Disneyland whenever she needed to get out of the house, and I would be around to run interference if necessary.

I took the job. I spent the first morning buying my tools and a hard hat, and reporting in to the Reinforcing Ironworkers Local to get my union card. That turned out to be a problem. Initially, they rejected my application because there were unemployed rodmen and they got first dibs. "You wanna take the food out of their kids' mouths and the shoes off their feet?" one guy asked nastily. *I got kids, too,* I thought but didn't say. When I was finally able to get a word in, I mentioned the Taft-Hartley Act and its right-to-work laws. "I have a job," I told them, "so you are required by law to give me membership in the union."

That comment didn't make me any friends.

I finally got to the jobsite at about two o'clock in the afternoon. I found the foreman and introduced myself. "I'm Norman," he said. "How in the hell did you get up here?"

"I walked up the stairs."

"Are you out of your mind? We're on the thirteenth floor! Why didn't you use the elevator?"

"Yeah, I know it's the thirteenth floor, I counted. I've never been in a construction elevator before," I admitted, "and I didn't see anyone around to show me how to operate it. I can't fly, so I took the stairs."

The rest of the day, I mostly carried rebar and did some tying. The next day, Norman sent me down to the ground floor where they were tying rebar for a bank vault. It was scheduled for a concrete pour in two days. The size and amount of rebar were unbelievable. I was assigned to work with an older pro named Ed, who told me, "You are to do nothing but tie, understood?" It was obvious to Ed that I was a greenhorn, so he took me under his wing. He showed me tricks of the trade to improve my speed, and for eight hours, I squeezed and cut wire with a nine-and-a-half-inch lineman's pliers. The next morning, I woke up in serious pain, my right hand cramped so tightly into a fist that I had to pry my fingers open. But we were finished with the bank vault by early afternoon the next day.

We headed up to the thirteenth floor—by elevator—to finish. Carrying twenty-foot #3 rebar raised hell on my shoulder, and dried blood had adhered my shirt to my skin. On the way home, I stopped at Newberry's and picked up a half dozen pot holders. I called my mother that evening. "Hey, Mom," I said. "Can you sew some pot holders inside the right shoulder of each of my work shirts?" No more bloody shoulders.

At the end of the second week, I was asked if I would like to take a swing-shift job working in a twelve-foot-diameter sewage tunnel near the Los Angeles airport. Union rules were that underground work paid a journeyman wage and night shifts got a 10 percent shift differential. That added up to $3.72 per hour, a 39 percent wage increase. Big money.

The tunnel was four miles long, so we had to take a tunnel train to get to the work area. The routine was to remove the train tracks where we were going to install the rebar, then we'd do the bottom first, then the sides, then set up scaffolding for the top. We tied an average of twenty tons of rebar per night. After a couple of weeks, during our eight p.m. "lunch" break, I suggested that we leave the train rails and set up scaffolding on a train car, do the ceiling first, the sides second, and then remove the rails and finish with the bottom. "That'll be more efficient," I said.

The foreman thought about it for a minute, then agreed to try it. The new routine saved so much time that two men got transferred to a day job, which cut their pay. They were not happy. At the end of the shift the following midnight, we were heading out of the tunnel when the train stopped suddenly. "Bryce," the foreman said, keeping his eyes focused forward, where the bright security lights in the security yard outside

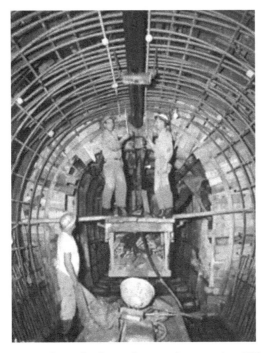

Los Angeles, twelve-foot outflow tunnel construction, 1958

illuminated the two men who had been reassigned. Each had a two-foot-long one-inch rebar in his hand. "Get off the train and wait in the tunnel." I did as told, moving silently down into the darkness.

"Where's Bryce?" one of the guys asked.

The foreman swore freely as he told them to get lost. "If you so much as put a foot on the jobsite again, I'll have you barred from the union. You'll never tie another rebar in Los Angeles County in your life, you hear me?"

I swallowed, waiting to see what would happen. Finally, the two guys left.

The foreman walked me to my car that night and drove behind me for a few miles to make sure I wasn't being followed. For the rest of the week, the train stopped to let me off before it exited the tunnel, and I waited while the foreman checked the yard. When the coast was clear, he walked me to my car and followed behind me.

The work was hard, but the money was good. Even better, I got to see my girls during the day before I left for work at three p.m. In early August, Joyce had morning sickness yet again. Baby number three was on his way.

FROM STUDENT TO TEACHER

I had one more year of school to go. I took all the classes to fulfill my chemistry major, including lots of math, plus a lot of other science classes. I took biology, botany, astronomy, geology, and physical geography. In a geology lab on minerals, I noticed one of the students was touching his tongue to every mineral. Why? He was looking for halite, crystallized sodium chloride, aka salt. After lab, I talked the lab assistant into a funny little prank: we dipped every mineral sample in a saturated solution of salt. We couldn't help laughing the next day at the look on the student's face when he tasted the minerals.

My physical geography class started at eight a.m., and, at the time, I was working the swing shift as a custodian at an elementary school in Phoenix. To add insult to injury, the professor was notoriously dull. To sprinkle a little more crystallized sodium chloride in the wound, he sat us alphabetically—there I was, in the middle of the front row, directly in front of him. Staying awake was absolute torture. He must've noticed, because on finals day, as he was passing out the test, he announced to the class, "Bryce has proven that you can learn while sleeping. He has only missed one question so far. It will be interesting to see how he does on the final." Lucky for me, he followed the textbook exactly. The one answer I'd missed previously was from a caption under a picture, and I'd learned my lesson. For the final, I read everything, including the captions. I aced it.

A child psychology class fulfilled the psychology requirement, and at the rate we were having kids, I could certainly use it. The professor lectured on developmental milestones, with a focus on preschool students' learning and behavior. Often, when she mentioned skills for these older kids, I'd chime in. "My daughter Vicki can do that," I'd say proudly. "She's only three!"

At some point, the professor finally had enough and pulled me aside after class one day. "Why don't you bring Vicki to my office," she said. The next week, I did just that. Later, the professor said that her lab/preschool was full, and that they had a long waiting list, but she would make an exception. "As long as you don't bring Vicki up in class anymore, OK?" she said.

Another graduation requirement was Introduction to Arts and Culture. I took two classes, which covered art, visual and stage; music, classic, opera, and jazz; dance, ballet and jazz; and architecture. We were assigned to go to art museums and the theater when possible, then write essays about our experiences. I'd thought I didn't need these classes because the Lyceum tickets my high school art and drama teacher had given me made me a convert, but it turned out that these two courses were the icing on the cake.

I had put off taking the required History 102 because I'd hated all the history courses thus far, from elementary through high school and History 101. All we'd done was memorize names, events, places, and dates. The very last semester, I resigned myself to another round of trying-to-stay-awake torture. But instead of History 102 being what I'd dreaded, it was a game changer. It was clear that the professor loved history, loved teaching, and loved storytelling. History wasn't set in stone, a boring list of "this happened, then that happened." It was about cause and effect! There were questions to be asked, mysteries to be solved! Why did some European colonizers settle near the shore, while others went inland? Perhaps it was the shape of the ships' hulls! What was a primary cause of the Protestant Reformation? The printing press!

With as many kids as I had, I thought I ought to take embryology. It was during my midterm exam, on March 28, 1959, that Joyce went into labor. Scott was born early the next morning, weighing seven pounds, six ounces.

I graduated that May, at the Sun Devil Stadium with over two thousand others. To ensure our attendance, the college set the cost of graduating in absentia at half again more than the fees plus the robe rental. There were too many of us to name, so they had us stand to receive our diplomas by group. With my fellow science majors, I stood to accept my bachelor of science degree. I was ready to go from student to teacher.

CHAPTER 8

Hi-Ho, It's Off to Work I Go

I hit the jackpot at the ASU career fair that spring of 1959. Seven high schools, six from Arizona and one from California, were looking for chemistry and/or physics teachers. They'd already received the portfolios prepared by the career services center for graduating students. Besides the standard materials—a photograph, a list of courses and extracurricular activities, grades, and a few sample essays—it included letters of recommendation, which students requested but were sent directly to the center without us knowing their contents. The letter of recommendation from my student teaching mentor must have been exceptionally good because five of the recruiters mentioned it when I was making the rounds. The recruiter from La Jolla said he was ready to offer me a teaching position solely based on that letter.

Five years later, I had an opportunity to read it. My mentor had written that after two weeks, he'd moved me from a regular chemistry class to his advanced class because I was a much better teacher than he was. My two years of teaching in the navy must have helped. I was floored by his generosity.

I applied for all seven high schools, and all seven high schools offered me a teaching position. Even though La Jolla offered the most money, the higher compensation didn't match the higher cost of living in that popular beach town, so I turned it down outright. I was most interested in Mesa High School—I had gone there my freshman and junior years, and I knew a lot of the teachers and already had a pool of friends there. During my interview with the superintendent, who had been my principal, I commented that I was surprised that he wanted me back after all the hell I had raised in my youth.

"There is nothing your students could do or think of doing that you haven't done or thought of doing," he said. "You'd be way ahead of them."

He was absolutely right. Unfortunately, Mesa High's overly packed teaching schedule and low salary were less than ideal.

Sunnyslope High School offered one of the best schedules and the second-best salary. To beat out the competition, the principal counted the two years that I had taught in the navy, thereby bumping me up to a third-year salary of $4,800. That was 26.3 percent more than what Mesa had offered. I did notice one odd stipulation in the contract: my job description included chairing the science department. I was only twenty-five, fresh out of college, and at least ten years younger than the rest of the faculty. On top of that, all but one of the teachers had taught at the school since its opening in 1953, making me the lowest person on the seniority totem pole. "Why me?" I asked the principal.

"You will be teaching the senior sciences, and you have taken courses in every science that we teach."

That went over like a lead balloon with my new coworkers. The only other drawback was that there were no fume hoods in the chemistry/physics lab. When I accepted the offer, the principal and I came to a verbal agreement that he would immediately have the fume hoods installed. I should have asked him to put that promise in writing.

LITTLE HOUSE ON THE CORNER

After signing my contract, Joyce and I went house hunting. We found a small starter house in north Phoenix on the corner of West Alice and North Third Avenues for $9,500. It was a thousand square feet, with three bedrooms, one and three-quarter baths, built out of concrete blocks. The outside was painted a light tan; the concrete floors were dyed oxblood red. An attached carport came with a laundry and storage room. An evaporative cooler, nicknamed "swamp cooler," was good enough for us—a window air-conditioner unit would have cost at least a month's salary and come with a monthly electric bill greater than the mortgage. Swamp coolers work by passing air from outside through water-saturated excelsior (aspen-wood fiber) pads, which causes the water to evaporate, lowering the temperature by around fifteen degrees while pushing warmer air out through the windows.

The living room in front and the dining room in back both had eight-foot picture windows. Sometimes birds would fly into them, then fall to the ground in a daze and, if left alone for a few minutes, get up, shake themselves off, and fly away again. Eventually I figured out that the other side of the windows was the best place for watching thunderstorms. Arizona is famous for these storms, especially during the summer and particularly in July, and there are more than half a million lightning strikes per year. Our backyard fence was the dividing line between our property and a church with a steeple topped by a lightning rod. The steeple was about 150 feet from our roofed back porch where, when we first moved in, I would sit to watch the lightning strike while Joyce corralled the kids inside. Once, I was doing just that, and suddenly, the hair on my arms stood up and I smelled the scent of ozone, a distinctly sweet, pungent smell, clean, like an electric spark. Then the lightning hit the rod with a zap. After that, whenever I felt static electricity, I would go inside to safely watch nature's light show through the window in the dining room or living room.

As our neighborhood was built upon a former citrus orchard, there were five grapefruit trees in our backyard and four Valencia orange trees in the front. Irrigation water rights came with the house; all of us in the neighborhood were allotted an amount equivalent to what the orchard had used. A one-foot berm surrounded all the yards, containing the eight to ten inches of water that flooded the lawns every two weeks, and once a month in the winter. I soon learned that citrus tree branches grow reaching toward the ground to protect their trunks from sunburn, and you have to trim them so that you can walk under the branches, then whitewash the trunks for sun protection. Like zucchinis in other parts of the world, the grapefruits all ripened at the same time, and we couldn't eat or drink the juice fast enough nor give them away. One afternoon, while driving by the Squirt Soda factory, it dawned on me that they might be interested in our citrus surplus. Lo and behold, they had a program that paid two dollars a crate. I signed up right away, and the money went to the kids for picking.

STARGAZING

Every time I brought up getting the fume hoods for the lab, the principal put me off, saying, "I'm trying to find the money." I continued to hound him, making sure he knew that I was keeping carbon copies of my requests to cover my butt.

The fourth Wednesday of the school year, a student thought

he was pulling a prank by plugging the vinyl tubing on another student's experiment. This caused chlorine gas to be released into the lab, and the pranked girl was rushed to the emergency room as a precaution. Thank goodness she was given a clean bill of health. Though every experiment had a safety section, clearly we needed another extra-intense lecture. Thursday was that lecture. Upon arriving to work the next Monday, I noticed that fume hoods had been installed over the weekend.

I think I learned more about teaching in my two years at Sunnyslope High than my students learned about science. The students and I had a great rapport, in no small part because of the closeness of our ages. To create professional distance, I wore dress shirts and ties, and every now and then, I mentioned my wife and kids. I arrived an hour before class and usually had students waiting for me, and I stayed for a couple of hours after school to help with homework, tutorials, and science club. Often, I had student company for the half-mile walk home.

The Soviets' launching of *Sputnik 1* on October 4, 1957, followed by the United States' *Explorer 1* on January 31, 1958, sparked a fascination with rockets. The science club had a subgroup of rocket enthusiasts, mostly physics students, who worked on design, with a few chemistry students, who tinkered with fuel formulas. We got permission to test and evaluate our rockets on the Luke Air Force Base practice range.

That spring of 1960, Jim Slipher, one of my chemistry students, invited me to meet his grandfather, Vesto Melvin Slipher, who was in town for a visit. A world-renowned astronomer who had been director of Lowell Observatory in Flagstaff, Arizona, for twenty-six years before his retirement in 1952, Dr. Slipher had received four honorary doctorate degrees and a handful of prizes for his work around the speed of the expansion of the universe. "Why don't you invite him to be a guest speaker for the science club?" I asked Jim.

At the end of Dr. Slipher's presentation, he said, "Mr. Bryce, you should bring the science club to Lowell Observatory so they can get a better view of the sky through our twenty-four-inch refractor telescope. Or the thirteen-inch that was used to discover Pluto in 1930!"

Uh-oh, I thought. As much as I would have loved to check out those telescopes myself, I didn't exactly need another task on my to-do list. I had three kids at home, and Joyce was pregnant again, with baby number four due in September. But the students would not let go of that invitation. While I hemmed and hawed, the club's officers selected a committee to plan the field trip, which, since it was a night experience, would have to be overnight.

On the way there, we visited two of the five national monuments near Flagstaff. We explored Montezuma Castle, a five-story dwelling in a sheer limestone cliff 90 feet above Beaver Creek, built by the Sinagua people between 1100 and 1425 CE, and Tuzigoot, a 110-room pueblo on top of a hill, built between 1000 and 1300 CE.

Two years earlier, Flagstaff had enacted the world's first outdoor lighting ordinance. (In 2001, the city would become the world's first International Dark Sky Place.) All lighting was aimed downward so that it would not interfere with Lowell Observatory's and the US Naval Observatory's combined thirty telescopes. That night, we could see a whole lot of stars.

After two hours of stargazing, we headed back to the hotel. The kids were amped up and not at all ready for bed, so I had to go around herding them into their rooms and quieting them down. While I was out kid-wrangling, three girls decided to pull a joke on me by "short-sheeting" my bed. Unbeknownst to them, Dick Stepan, the other chaperon, was sharing my room. He'd left the door unlocked for me and gone straight to bed; the girls entered, closed the door, and flipped on the light.

"What the—" Mr. Stepan shouted, sitting up in his blue-striped pajamas.

"Oh!" gasped one of the girls. "We thought this was Mr. B's room!"

"Sorry we woke you up," said another as they turned and fled, giggling.

Once I finally got everyone settled, I went to my room, more than ready to hit the hay. I was surprised to find Dick awake. "So," he said, then filled me in on what had happened. *I hope this doesn't get around the school,* I thought. *Sure doesn't look good.*

The next day, we visited the Wupatki ruins, a multistory Sinagua pueblo with more than one hundred rooms built out of red flagstone. It was built on a hill between 1040 and 1100 CE, right after the eruption of Sunset Crater, a 1,120-foot cinder cone that spewed ash for miles, enriching the soil and attracting Native farmers. The lava formed tunnels big enough to walk through, which the students were thrilled to do. The last stop was Walnut Canyon and the alcoves below its rim, built by forming walls of stone around limestone caves.

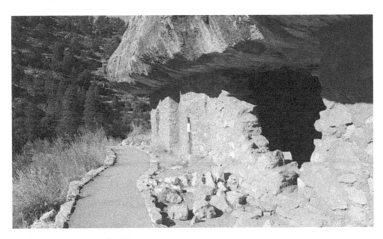

Walnut Canyon cave dwellings

Except for the attempted short-sheeting drama, the field trip was a resounding success. Soon after, a group of students approached me to ask if I would teach an advanced chemistry course. I took the request to the principal, who initially wanted to veto it. "You'd have to drop one of your classes," he said, "and it would be a small class and not pay for itself." Without giving it a lot of thought, I volunteered to teach it as an extra course. "I won't drop anything," I promised, "as long as I can restrict the class size to ten students. And I select the students."

"All right," the principal said. "I'll see if I can scrape together four hundred dollars for you."

I should have known he was not a good scraper after his foot-dragging over the fume hoods, and I never did see that four hundred dollars. And I accepted two more students than I'd agreed to—what a pushover I was. Still, it was the best class that I had ever taught. The students were all seniors, and most of them were taking physics and advanced math as well.

Eleven of the twelve went on to college. Lucy, the only one who did not, was extremely bright, a straight-A student who loved science and learned quick as lightning. I knew that she would need financial aid to go to college, so I took it upon myself to reach out to my academic advisor and mentor, Dr. Brown. With his help, I got a scholarship for her at ASU.

I made a big mistake by not talking with her first. Excited by my successful string pulling, I called up her father. "She's not going to college," he told me. "We need her here to support the family."

I was embarrassed and dismayed in equal measure. Anyway, she didn't need me, after all—she eventually got a job in a lab, working her way up until she was doing work that normally required a BS degree. Later I heard that both of her sons have biochemistry PhDs. If my source is correct, nine of the eleven other students earned doctorate degrees.

UP, UP, AND AWAY

Susan was born on September 5, 1960. The same OB-GYN who had delivered Bonnie and Scott delivered her, mainly because Joyce thought he was great, but also because he extended his flat fee of fifty dollars per child. That was worth the thirty-mile drive from Phoenix to the hospital in Mesa. Susan was the biggest of our babies, at eight pounds, three ounces, and she had the darkest complexion and coal-black hair that, over time, grew out blond.

My second year at Sunnyslope passed in the blink of an eye. The science club and the advanced chemistry class on top of my regular course load, the grading and the lab prep, plus three kids and a baby and wife who was, once again, pregnant—when, exactly, did I sleep? I really can't remember.

In the spring, I received a scholarship from the National Science Foundation for a graduate program for science teachers at ASU. The grant would not only pay for tuition and supplies; it included living expenses, which, with four kids and one on the way, was a lot of dough, a much better deal than what I got as a teacher at Sunnyslope High. We stayed in the house on the former citrus grove during the school year and summer that it took for me to earn my master's degree. Kevin was born that fall, on November 22, 1961. He was the smallest of the bunch, at seven pounds, two ounces. But for what he lacked in size, he made up for in energy. He was in perpetual motion.

I had enjoyed teaching the advanced chemistry class at Sunnyslope so much that, once I'd completed the program, I applied to community colleges and small four-year colleges as well as high schools. I sent out thirteen inquiries and got eleven replies of interest. Joyce and I went over the pluses and minuses of each, assessing location, salary, cost of living, teaching schedule, benefits, student body size, and public versus private as the criteria to make our first cut.

While we still dreamed of returning to the Pacific Northwest, after a phone interview with Whidbey Island's high school principal, I removed it from the list. The schedule was so ridiculous it was funny. The principal had told me that, because of the small enrollment size, I would be teaching general science, biology, chemistry on odd years and physics on even years, algebra, and geometry. That was five preparations a day. Then, to top it off, he added, "I noticed that you played football. We'd pay you extra to be the assistant football coach."

"Anything else I can do?" I asked sarcastically. I think he must have figured he'd lost me because he replied, "You could drive the school bus."

Need I say more?

Soon after that call, I crossed the two Oregon colleges off my list. The first, Southern Oregon University, had wanted me to teach more math than chemistry. The second, George Fox University in Newberg, looked promising until the president said the job was mine and my name was being sent to the board of regents to sign off. The next day, he called back to ask if I was a Quaker or evangelical Christian. "Neither," I said. I received a letter to confirm the withdrawal of the school's offer the following week.

By this time, I was down to four two-year colleges in California: Santa Barbara City College, Ventura College, Grossmont College, and Citrus College. I drove west for the face-to-face interviews. I will never forget my interview with the president of Santa Barbara, who was the spitting image of actor Edward G. Robinson: short and bald with a shiny forehead and a big cigar hanging out of the corner of his mouth. After our introductions, he said, "If you're such a damn good chemist, then why aren't you working for a big company and making big money, instead of applying for a teaching job at a two-year college?"

I was caught off guard. When I didn't answer right away,

he turned his palm up and extended it toward me, as if to say, *I'm waiting.* That did it. I swallowed and then launched into a reply while trying to keep my cool. When I finally shut up, a grin spread across his face and he puffed out a cloud of smoke. "That's what I wanted to hear," he said. "You are a man with a passion for teaching, not one of those who can't do, so teach."

Before accepting his offer, Joyce and I checked out Santa Barbara. It was beautiful but clearly inhabited by the wealthy, with those who worked for them commuting in. I couldn't stand the idea of driving thirty miles every morning and evening, so that was a no-go. Next, I turned down Grossmont because it was so new that the campus was still on the drawing board, and classes were held in the evenings at a nearby high school. Ventura was a maybe, but the interview was so casual that I wondered if the science department would be up to snuff, and the housing situation wasn't great, either. Citrus College it was. To quote my dad: "You always find what you're looking for the last place you look."

With that, we sold our Sunnyslope house for $12,000 and moved to Glendora, California.

CHAPTER 9

California, Here We Come

It was a beautiful spring day, the morning after a light April rain that had washed the smog out of the air. Joyce and I were headed to Citrus College for the last of our list of interviews. As we exited Interstate 10, a strip of road built in 1935 and called the Ramona Freeway by locals, onto Grand Avenue, the windshield was filled with a breathtaking view of the San Gabriel Mountains. It had been a wet spring, and the mountains were covered with a blanket of green underneath crystal-clear skies. It seemed as though Mother Nature was doing her best to sell us on the area.

We were more than an hour early, so we took ourselves on a self-guided tour of the town of Glendora and the neighborhood near the college. Incorporated in 1911, this quaint suburb twenty-six miles east of Los Angeles had a population of twenty-five thousand, and the commercial area was made up of mostly privately owned stores and shops.

The college campus was a mix of old buildings and new

construction. Enrollment had recently exploded (it was 982 students in 1959, and by 1965, it would be 5,535), the fastest and largest increase in the fifty years since the school was founded in 1915. There was a lot of construction on the west side of campus; the east side was beautifully landscaped, filled with plants in bloom. Flowering pear trees lined the sidewalk west of the chemistry and earth science building. Later I learned that nearby Monrovia Nursery coveted those trees, and that they had agreed to prune the trees every year so that they could use the cuttings for grafting. In exchange, they had donated camellia plants to the college. All around campus were the blossoming camellia shrubs, their flowers snow white, showstopping magenta, and soft blush.

I was surprised to find the president's office in a portable. Dr. Glenn Vaniman explained that it was more important that the new buildings be used for educating students than for administration. I liked that kind of thinking. He, Vice President Merlin Eisenbise, and I had a great interview. I was impressed with both men and thought they would be great to work for. Afterward, Dr. Vaniman and Dr. Eisenbise walked me outside. "Take your wife to lunch and get acquainted with Glendora," said Dr. Eisenbise, "then come back at one o'clock. Oh, and please do bring your wife, we would like to meet her."

I left with the feeling that I was going to be offered a contract. Joyce and I had pastrami sandwiches at The Hat, then headed north on Grand Avenue up the mountain to get a view of the valley below. A brown cloud of exhaust hovered over the freeway. Little did we know that on a windy day, not only would that cloud reach our house, it would block our view of the mountaintops.

On our way back down, I noticed the construction of several new homes at the end of a couple side streets, and since we had some time before our appointment back at the school, I turned the car down one of the streets to investigate. I stopped in front of a house-in-progress and rolled down my window to talk to a man who appeared to be the foreman. "When will the houses be for sale?" I asked.

"I'm guessing end of May, maybe first week of June," he said.

At the meeting, the president and vice president did offer a contract and went about detailing the advantages of the college to Joyce. The Community Education program had classes in graphic arts, printmaking, ceramics, and sculpture, Dr. Eisenbise told her, as well as theater, performance, scene and costume design, writing and poetry, music vocal and instrumental—the list went on. "On Saturdays, there is live theater and symphonies for the public," Dr. Vaniman added. Then the two men turned to me.

I would be teaching two chemistry classes, a total of six hours of lecture and twelve hours in the lab per week; I would be making 40 percent more than I did at Sunnyslope and teaching seven hours less. I tried not to show my glee—I was ready to sign, but Joyce and I needed to talk it over first. "Oh, and Herb?" Dr. Vaniman added. "Because of our rapid growth, we're going to hire a second chemist as soon as we can. When he comes aboard, you and he can negotiate who will teach what."

I glanced at Joyce, who was looking relaxed, like someone who'd spent a day free of her five young kids—my mother was minding them at my folks' place in La Mirada—with a good lunch in her belly, surrounded by flowers. "We need to check out the prices of homes in the area," I said.

"Take a week to think it over," Dr. Eisenbise told us.

The four of us shook hands, and then Joyce and I found a bench under the shade of a big cork oak tree. The first thing she said was "I was ready to hand you a pen. I love this town."

"I do, too."

"Didn't the man say those houses would be available by June?"

I nodded. "Let's drive back up and see if we can find out how to get ahold of the contractor."

The foreman was talking with a man wearing a carpenter's belt when we pulled up. I got out and headed over to ask how to contact someone about buying a house.

He turned and pointed to a few houses in various stages of construction. "There's a bunch for sale now at the north end of the street. Go to the first house on the right on the corner—the garage is being used as the sales office. Someone should be there. If not, there should be sales info available."

"Thank you."

"Good luck! We build great houses. Hope you find what you need."

The Realtor, Melvin, was there, and he showed us around. We were very impressed. The houses were priced based on the number of bedrooms and lot size. Those at the end of the cul-de-sac had much bigger lots, and the price for a four-bedroom was $19,500. This was well within our price range.

We took ourselves on another tour of the house without him and discussed the contract. Joyce was excited to leave Phoenix. She wanted out of the heat. We both loved Glendora and the location, and the new houses were within walking distance of the college. It would be a good place for the kids, too. I felt it was the best of all the offers, and she agreed. "Let's sign it," she said.

On the way to the car, I poked my head into the sales office. "Melvin, how long are you going to be here?"

"Till six."

"We'll be back before you leave."

At the college, I asked the secretary (yes, that was her title, this was 1962) if the president or vice president were available, and she said that they were in a meeting. I handed her the signed contract and turned to leave. "Wait a minute," she said, standing up from behind her desk and knocking on the door to the president's office before opening it. I could see four people inside. She went in and whispered to Dr. Eisenbise while handing him my contract. He got up and came out.

"I'm excited to be working with you," he said, shaking my hand.

"Thanks. Me, too. We're leaving tomorrow, got to get back to ASU for class on Monday. But we'll be back in June to buy a house."

"I'll see you in June," he said.

NO BACKING OUT NOW

On our way back to La Mirada, we discussed our favorite of the houses, which was twice the size of the one we were living in Phoenix and came with a built-in stove and double oven, plus a matching fridge. Would Melvin keep his word about letting us buy it while we were still living in Phoenix? We talked ourselves into staying in California for another day to see if we could buy it before we left.

We were at the sales office by ten a.m. "No need for a sales pitch," I told Melvin. "We're here to go over the sale agreement and read the fine print. What's the down payment?"

"Either one of you a veteran?"

"I am. Navy."

"Down payment will be fifteen hundred dollars."

"Don't sell it while we're gone."

We found a bank in downtown Glendora. We met the bank's branch president. I told him I'd just signed a contract to teach at Citrus College, and we'd already found a house we wanted to buy. "I want to take out a loan," I said.

"For the mortgage?"

"No. For the down payment. I just need it till I get back to Phoenix."

He held up an index finger, picked up the phone, and dialed. "Glenn, it's James. I have a young man by the name of Herb Bryce in my office. Says he signed a contract to teach chemistry at the college." Pause. "Yeah, OK. Says he wants to buy a house just above La Fetra School." Pause. "OK, thanks, Glenn. Bye-bye." He replaced the receiver and smiled. "I'm on the board of regents for Citrus College," he said. "Just checking with Dr. Vaniman. He told me to help you buy the house so you won't back out of the contract."

"Great."

"But," he said, holding up an index finger again, "the bank doesn't loan money for down payments." Joyce and I glanced at each other. This was going to be a problem. "There is another option," he continued. "Do you think it will cost at least that much to move?"

I caught on quickly. "Sure, at least that much. Maybe more!"

He excused himself, walked over to a teller, and returned with a sheet of paper. "Please fill out this loan request." The teller followed a few minutes later with a check for $1,500.

Joyce and I took it to the sales office, checked that the address was 611 West Whitcomb Avenue, and signed all the papers.

My mother was on cloud nine when she heard the news. No backing out now.

ANOTHER BIG MOVE

A second cousin of mine owned a real estate company, and when we told him that we were moving to California, he bought our house in Phoenix for $12,000, no fees. He said he would make his profit when he sold it. Melvin called in mid-May to give us an update on how the house was coming along. "Looks like you will be able to move in June 11. Landscaping is scheduled for the week of the Fourth. They'll put on the finishing coat of stucco next week. While it's drying, my guys will paint the trim, install the light fixtures and doorknobs, and put down the linoleum and carpet."

I finished graduate school in early June. I had been helping Grant move bees and extract honey, and I told him that I would work for free for a week if he would help us move and let us use his truck, then drive it back, which would save me two trips. After we put the stake-bed sides on, we loaded the truck and covered it with a tarp to protect the furniture. The area between Indio and Whitewater has sandstorms so hellacious that they've been known to sandblast windshields and strip paint off cars, as my dad learned firsthand in 1949. He was coming home to Fontana from a visit to relatives in Mesa, and when he arrived, it looked like Mother Nature had taken sandpaper to the windshield. We took the extra precaution because, even though we'd be warned if the wind was picking up—insurance companies wouldn't cover sandstorms—better safe than sorry.

We left on Thursday so we could meet with Melvin on Friday morning to go over in detail what was left to do. Joyce asked if we could see inside the house. "The cabinets are being installed and the doors are getting hung," Melvin said, "but if you come back at four fifteen, I'll give you a tour."

We arrived a little after three o'clock and parked in front of our house. A truck loaded with bags of finishing stucco and a forklift were dropping off pallets at each of the eight houses on the street. I checked the bags in front of our house; the stucco wasn't the color we'd picked out. Once they'd stopped at the next house, I walked over to the guy supervising the process. "I think you made a mistake," I said. He looked at his clipboard.

"That's what we were given," he told me. I waited for them to leave, then examined the piles at the other houses. The third one I looked at had "our" color.

Melvin pulled up as the last of the workers left. Joyce had never been in a house during construction and was surprised to see electrical wire sticking out of the ceiling and walls, and cupboards sitting on the floor in the middle of the living room. After he left, I told her that I wanted to exchange the bags of stucco. I hopped in our Volkswagen bus and got to work, switching the piles of thirty eighty-pound bags of finishing stucco. I lifted more than two tons—good thing I was only twenty-eight at the time.

We moved in a week later. The kids and, more importantly, Joyce were thrilled with all the space. The front of the house was professionally landscaped, but the back was nothing but dirt, so I spent the summer landscaping the backyard and building the kids a playhouse fort. By the time school began, we were all settled in.

STARTING MY NEW JOB WITH A BANG

I started work at Citrus College two weeks before the fall term of 1962. I needed to check the lab drawers and supply room and order anything we were out of, to double-check that there were fume hoods—there were—and to work on the first week's lectures and demonstrations. The school had hired Ron Levy, an organic chemist who was the perfect match for me, an analytical and physical chemist. He had two PhDs, one in chemistry and one in philosophy, and he was fun to boot, with the rare skill of being able to talk about topics other than chemistry, a definite bonus when you're sharing an office.

Tuesday, the second day of class, was a lab day. The experiment was simple, and meant to illustrate the different ways, chemical and physical, to separate the elements sulfur and iron. One of the methods required the use of carbon disulfide. "Dispose of all carbon disulfide in this lidded crock," I told the class, looking around the room to make sure they were listening. "Do *not*—I repeat, do *not*—pour it down the sink drain. Carbon disulfide is flammable and can explode if you get the right mixture of fumes and oxygen. Understood?"

Nods all around. Of course, more than one student did not follow directions, and the sink in the lecture hall demonstration table had a dry P trap because it had not been used all summer. That afternoon, I walked by the lecture hall and saw a student leaning over his chemistry book with a lit cigarette in his mouth. I poked my head in the door. "Hey!" I said. "No smoking in the building."

The student shrugged and, before I could stop him, flicked his cigarette into the sink.

There was a tremendous explosion, and the building was immediately filled with carbon dioxide and sulfur dioxide fumes pouring out of every drain in every room. Out of the women's restroom shuffled a student, her panties around her ankles and her skirt soaked. "The toilet exploded!" she cried.

"Step out of your panties and get out of the building as fast as you can!" I yelled.

Dr. Levy came out of the men's restroom just down the hall, the front of his shirt and pants drenched. He must have had some idea of what had happened, because as he headed out the door, he commented nonchalantly, "I've peed in a lot of urinals in my life, but this is the first one that peed on me."

A PREGNANCY, A CON MAN, THEN ME

Sometime during that first year, I learned the reason for the position at Citrus becoming available in August, which is the worst time to recruit a sciences instructor, chemistry in particular. (In academics, faculty recruiting normally takes place in April.)

The year prior, a student who was obviously pregnant approached the vice president to ask how she could find the chemistry instructor. "I need help paying the doctor and hospital expenses," she told him. The instructor's resignation suddenly left the science department without a chemistry instructor for the coming year, and the college put out an emergency ad for a chemist. They received a glowing application—perhaps a little too glowing—but it was so close to the start of the semester that they hired someone (I'll call him Mr. Con) without properly checking his references.

Turned out that Mr. Con had never taken a chemistry class. The other faculty caught on that he was not teaching at the level he should have been. They reported it and sent students to the VP for instruction to complain. But Mr. Con was a good con man, liked by nonscience faculty and staff, and it took until halfway through the second semester before the VP relented.

That's when I was hired to replace Mr. Con. He'd left without cleaning out his desk or file cabinet in his office, and I made the unhappy discovery that all his tests were true or false, and his lecture notes made it obvious that he was only one page ahead of the students.

Oh boy.

I was not surprised that my Chem 102 students were struggling. Had they learned anything in Chem 101? On the Monday of the second week, we talked for nearly an hour about the previous semester, and I found out that Mr. Con had bribed the students into taking Chem 102 by not requiring them to take the Chem 101 final exam if they signed up for it. It was a small class of about twenty students, and our lectures were on Mondays, Wednesdays, and Fridays, with the three-hour lab on Thursdays. "How about we meet on Tuesdays, too?" I suggested. "We'll fit in Chem 101 and Chem 102 so that you get what you paid for."

IF IT'S RED, IT'S A COMMIE

One afternoon, I got a panicked call from the librarian. "Herb!" she said, her voice an octave higher than usual. "Can you come help me?" My office was the closest one to the library, and when I arrived a minute later, the librarian was having a yelling match and a trash-barrel tug-of-war with an elderly woman.

"Whoa!" I said, stepping between them and holding up my hands. "What's going on here?"

"Look!" the librarian said, gesturing to the barrel. "This woman is throwing books with red covers into the trash!"

I glanced down, and, indeed, the trash can was filled with red-covered books.

"OK, all right. Why don't you both let go of the barrel and take one step back so we can talk?" To my surprise, they did what I asked. "Good. OK," I said, turning to the older woman. "Please explain what you are doing."

"I'm clearing out all the Communist books!" she said, her face flushed.

"Ah," I said. At that time, Orange County was a hot spot for "John Birchers"—members of the John Birch Society, a right-wing anti-Communist organization named after a US Army Intelligence specialist killed by Chinese Communists while serving in Anhui in 1945. I reached into the barrel and pulled out a book. "This is a book on biological evolution." I showed her the front cover, pointing to the title, *Phylogenetics*. "It has nothing to do with communism."

"It's a Communist book, it has a red cover!" she insisted. "When you see red, you think of communism!"

It was hard to argue with that. I finally convinced her to
allow me to escort her off campus. Outside the library, we
walked by a puzzled custodian. "Looking for your trash barrel?" I said. "It's in there."

As we passed a camellia bush loaded with red flowers
near the edge of campus, I couldn't help myself. I picked one
and handed it to her, chuckling. *Here's a Communist flower,* I
thought as she thanked me.

CLOSING THE GAP

In the fall of my second year at Citrus College, I got a call
from the president of the Southern California section of the
American Chemical Society (ACS). The ACS wanted to start
a two-year college committee, and he was looking for four or
five two-year chemistry instructors to organize it. Once the
committee was formed, we launched another committee in
the national ACS, and the chemistry professor at El Camino
College, Bill Mooney, chaired both.

At the end of that semester, I was startled by the drop-
out rate and the number of students who'd received D and F
grades. I checked with Dr. Levy. "I'm sorry to say that a lot of
the kids failed," he told me. We agreed that this was not acceptable, we needed to do something about it. I took the lead
on the problem. We surveyed other two- and four-year colleges to find that they were having the same problem. Why?
Because of the gap between high school and college chemistry
courses.

This gap was widening because science was advancing,
and teaching requirements were decidedly not. Approximately
75 percent of high school chemistry teachers did not have
degrees in chemistry. The majority had taken three classes
in chemistry; some had taken only one or two classes. Most

states allowed principals to make emergency hires for science classes, and often the teacher would stay on in that assignment for lack of better options. Chemistry teaching positions were lucky to get three or four applicants, whereas jobs in the English department got three or four hundred.

Meanwhile, the beeps heard on the radio around the world on October 4, 1957, had woken up American politicians. The Soviet Union had beat us. They'd launched Earth's first satellite, *Sputnik 1*, a twenty-two-inch-diameter ball that weighed 184 pounds. American scientists had been caught with their pants down. We'd been counting on Wernher von Braun and his group of German rocket scientist team leaders who, in 1944, realized that Germany would lose World War II and so surrendered to the Americans. They'd been sent to Fort Bliss, Texas. For fifteen years, they worked on rockets and ballistic missiles for the US Army's military top-secret Operation Paperclip. With the help of these German scientists, we'd answered the Soviet Union by launching *Explorer 1*, a thirty-pound, eighty-inch-long, and six-and-a-quarter-inch-diameter satellite, on January 31, 1958. The Cold War was heating up, and the American government called for more scientists. On top of that, the huge instrumental advancements in the mid-twentieth century allowed biologists to discover and analyze molecular and metabolic pathways of the cell like the Krebs cycle and glycolysis. Biochemistry and bioengineering became front and center in the sciences, which, in turn, widened the gap between high school and college chemistry.

Nobel laureate Glenn T. Seaborg acquired a grant from the National Science Foundation to form a steering committee to determine how to close this gap. They produced CHEM Study, a curriculum and textbook that would accomplish this, and which would be used across the nation so that all American students learned the same thing. Meanwhile, at Reed College, another group was developing the Chem Bond program, which was the more rigorous of the two and the one to which I contributed. Ultimately, CHEM Study won out.

We concluded that we could not rely on all of the students having the proper background, so we developed a prep course for those who did not pass the science major chemistry entrance exam. The drop-out rate and failures almost disappeared. It was a huge success.

UPGRADES

When the division chair resigned and moved to San Luis Obispo to help start Cuesta College, Dr. Ron Levy, the oldest science teacher and the most educated, was rightfully named physical and earth sciences division chair. Turned out that he did not want the position, however, and at his request, I kept the budget and ordered supplies. After a couple of months, Ron asked me to come with him to the president's office. On the way, he said that he was going to resign as division chair and ask that I get the position instead. "You are doing all the work, you should have the title," he said.

This gave me the credibility to write grants and develop programs. The chem department had only three double-pan analytical balances, which made quantitative analysis lab work awfully slow for twenty-four students. Items to be weighed went on one pan; you placed weights on the other pan until the two pans were in balance. Trying to get the correct combinations of weights can take a long time, up to fifteen or twenty minutes per sample, and when you have three samples that need to be weighed at least twice, you spend a lot of time using the balance. Mettler had a new electronic balance that would give the weight to the fourth decimal place, one-ten-thousandth of a gram (approximately the equivalent of the weight of your fingerprint), in ten seconds. I worked with our chemical supply salesman and Mettler and got two free Mettler balances for every one the college bought. We bought three and ended up with nine.

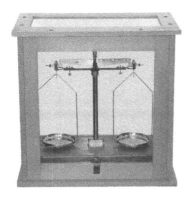

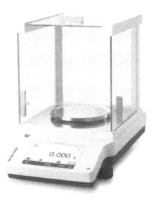

Double-pan analytical balance   *Mettler electronic balance*

My next grant was for a planetarium. We got a Spitz projector with a twenty-four-foot dome and seating for seventy-two people. It opened in 1965, and we needed someone to operate it. As I was negotiating with the vice president about this, one of the college math instructors approached me and said that he had worked for a planetarium and would love to operate this one. Besides being used for classes, it was open to the public one night a week. It became so popular that we had to issue passes.

The next big project was the new physical science building. After all the planning I did with architects, however, I would not get to teach in it.

That spring at the national ACS meeting, Bill Mooney and I were talking when the president of the national ACS happened to walk by. Bill stopped the ACS president and told him that he had been offered a dean of instruction position and he would need to resign as chair of the two-year committee. The president asked if he knew of anyone who could take over. Bill pointed at me and said, "Herb can. He helped get the committee started."

To the Chem Ed division for the national ACS, I wrote a letter describing our program for closing the gap between high school and college chemistry, and asking for a session on the problem. He took me up on it. I ended up giving sessions to both two-year and four-year colleges about our program twice a year for the next two years.

Being the chair of the national two-year education committee and giving these sessions in the committee got me noticed and enlarged my circle of contacts throughout the United States.

In the spring of 1966, I turned up the driveway, the very last board to finish the retaining wall in our backyard in the back of the car. It was a regular glorious California afternoon, with blue skies and flowers in bloom. Joyce was standing in front of the house, waving her arms and jumping up and down. As I parked, I saw the note pinned to her blouse—sticky notes had not been invented yet.

"Dr. Larry Blake, dean of instruction of Seattle Central College, called!" she said as soon as I opened the car door. She'd fallen in love with the Pacific Northwest when we lived there, and a job offer in Seattle was an answer to her prayers.

"But Seattle doesn't have a community college," I said, confused.

"Here," she said, unpinning the note and handing it to me. "The dean said they are starting one and they want you to come up and put together the science department. He wants you to call him as soon as you can."

"Slow down," I said. "Let me see what they're offering." I didn't want to rain on her parade, but I had to remind her that I'd signed a contract with Citrus College the previous week to teach the coming year. "Let's get the facts, then we'll talk it over, OK? If we really want to go to Seattle, then I'll have to ask Dr. Vaniman if I can get out of my contract."

After the call with Dr. Blake, I was ready to take the job; Joyce did not need to talk me into it. The offer was for me to be division chair of sciences, which would entail me setting up the science department and teaching chemistry. My salary would be a third more than what I'd be earning at Citrus.

I wasn't too eager to tell Dr. Vaniman, but knew I needed to get it over with so he had as much time as possible to find my replacement.

The camellias were as bright as they had been when I'd first arrived on campus four years earlier, lining the walkways with whites and pinks and Communist reds. I'd miss those flowers, but I felt like I needed more opportunities to grow, and I wanted to live in a place that wasn't redlined to keep out Latino and Black people. I knew I was making the right decision as I told the president about my conversation with Dr. Blake.

"Sounds like you are excited about the offer," he said. "You would be crazy not to take it."

I breathed out a sigh of relief, then took a deep breath, preparing to bring up the main issue.

"I know what you're going to say, Herb. We can void your contract, don't worry about that. I'd love for you to continue here, but if I try to hold you to your contact, your heart wouldn't be a hundred percent with Citrus. Good luck in Seattle."

CHAPTER 10

Seattle, the Gateway to the Pacific Northwest

The Evergreen State captured our hearts when Joyce and I lived on Whidbey Island during my last two years in the navy. Both of us had grown up in the desert, and though Washingtonians complained about the interminable rain, we enjoyed it. We loved the Puget Sound and Skagit Bay and the islands to the north, the ferry ride on choppy dark-gray waters. We loved the evergreen trees and the year-round lushness, the ever-present dampness in the air that made every breath fresh and full. We had often talked about moving back after I finished college, but with each new job in Arizona and Southern California, and with each new mouth to feed, we'd put it off. Now we were answering the call of the Pacific Northwest. I had accepted a job in Seattle, a dynamic city surrounded by the ultimate in natural beauty.

In the summer of 1966, Joyce and I drove up to Seattle to find a house to rent. Little did we know that Boeing was hiring locally as well as out of state, and therefore we'd have a lot of competition for decent housing. Just a few months earlier, the company had announced that they were going to build the 747 airliner, and, in April, Pan Am had ordered twenty-five of these aircraft for a cost of $525 million. This was a monumental engineering and management challenge, and Boeing set about hiring thousands of workers. They needed a building big enough to meet the demand, and pronto, and so the company began constructing one of the biggest buildings in the world, its size equivalent to forty football fields. The location? Everett, Washington, about thirty miles north of Seattle's Capitol Hill neighborhood where I would be teaching.

What we thought would take two or three days turned out to take ten days. While house hunting, we stayed at the Roosevelt Hotel in downtown Seattle. When the newspaper hit the street in the morning, I was there, waiting at the newsstand. At first, I was polite and waited until nine a.m. to call the number in the "For Rent" listings. The answer was always "I'm sorry, it's been rented." So I started calling earlier. By the tenth day, I was calling at six a.m.

"Good morning," I said groggily. The first question the equally groggy man on the other end of the line asked was "You work for Boeing?"

"No," I answered. "I'm a college professor. I'll be starting at Seattle Central in September." I don't know if he liked the idea of having a college instructor as a tenant better than a Boeing employee, but he sounded pleased with my answer. We exchanged information, and he told me to meet him at the rental in Lake Forest Park at eight.

I had no idea where Lake Forest Park was, and it would be twenty-seven years before the advent of GPS. Joyce and I asked the hotel clerk for directions and made it with time to spare. The owner hadn't arrived yet, but a group of eager would-be renters was already waiting. Lake Forest Park, it turned out, was about halfway between Capitol Hill and the new airplane factory. Needless to say, my heart sank. When the owner did arrive, everyone started bidding on the house, sight unseen. I looked at Joyce and shrugged. "Oh well," I said. "We'll find something one of these days."

Then the owner called out, "Who are the Bryces?" Joyce and I raised our hands. "Come with me," he said.

The house needed some work. A couple of the bedrooms in the basement were framed but not finished. The owner pointed out a stack of plywood panels. "I'll move those out before the renters move in," he said. With that, I saw my opportunity. "If you leave the paneling," I told him, "I would be happy to install the electrical and panel the rooms before my job starts in September." That clinched it.

When we got back outside, the owner announced to the group that the house had been rented. They left, muttering under their breath and giving us the stink eye. By the end of July, we'd signed a one-year lease—which, we hoped, would give us time to find a place to buy—and moved into the five-bedroom house, which I fixed up as promised.

On the whole, the kids took the move well. The only grumbling came from sixth-grader Vicki, who complained about her new school's dress code that did not allow girls to wear pants. "My legs freeze while I'm waiting for the bus!" she said. Even so, she insisted on wearing her beloved black patent leather Mary Jane shoes that she'd worn in California. We tried to talk her into getting saddle oxford shoes, but it wasn't until she'd stood in the rain every morning for a couple of weeks that she gave in.

A FARM FOR THE KIDS

The next year, we bought a parcel of wooded land bordered by Fifteenmile Creek, just south of Issaquah. This was a more rural area back then, over the floating I-90 bridge past Mercer Island, on the other side of Lake Washington.

Designing the house was a family project. First, I built a "garage" for us to live in while the house was under construction. In reality, it was a small cabin of about one thousand square feet, with a concrete floor and a front wall designed to be easily removed when it was time to install the two-car garage door. There was a three-quarter bath and a rudimentary space we used as a kitchen, which would become my workshop. We slept on a mezzanine-level floor separated into three sleeping spaces, one for the parents, one for the girls, and one for the boys.

We agreed that the house should overlook the creek. Joyce wanted an art studio with space for a 240-volt kiln. I needed a small office. I asked the kids if they'd rather have two big dormitory-style rooms or small single bedrooms. They voted for each having their own bedroom. We ended up with a 3,330-square-foot house. It was designed to reduce cost, though I did have to hire some subcontractors because we were working on a steep slope, and I didn't have the proper equipment or the experience for building retaining walls, footers, and foundations. Two offset three-story towers were connected by a staircase, and tongue-and-groove subflooring made up the ceiling for the floor below. I bought lumber by the foot to minimize waste, and I did as much of the labor as I could, with the help of Kevin, who mainly helped me lay the hardwood floors, keeping me supplied with boards and nails. The two thousand square feet of the bottom two floors were covered with short (eight to eighteen inches long) and narrow (one and three fourth inches wide) oak. The top flooring, one thousand square feet, was hardwood planks.

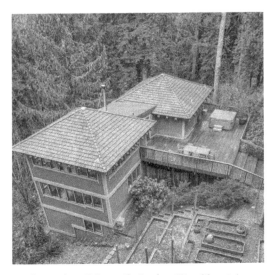

Our house above Fifteenmile Creek on Tiger Mountain

When surveyed, our five acres turned out to be only four, but since we'd bought it by the parcel and not by the acre, we didn't get a fifth of the cost back. At least the tax bill was reduced by a fifth. The kids couldn't have cared less about that missing acre—they thought we'd bought a farm. (When I tried to tell them about my grandparents' real farm in Arizona, however, their eyes glazed over.) Right away, they started requesting livestock. Vicki wanted a horse to ride, Bonnie wanted white rabbits to breed, and Susan wanted a Nankin bantam rooster and hen as pets—she loved the dark-red coloring and black tail, plus, she thought baby chicks were cute. Aspiring carpenter and entrepreneur Kevin wanted to go into the egg business. Scott was the only one who wasn't interested in animal husbandry, probably because I'd pulled no punches when telling the kids that if they had animals, they would be responsible for taking care of them.

Kevin asked for twenty-four chickens to get the ball rolling, and when I called a hatchery to see about buying baby chicks, they gave me a price of more than $2,000. I gasped. "You're kidding! Right?"

"That's a good price," the gravelly voice said. "It's eighty-five dollars per thousand."

I chuckled. "I think you misunderstood me," I said. "I want to buy *two dozen* baby chicks for my son. He wants to raise chickens so he can sell the eggs."

"Oh, I see. Well, we normally sell by the thousands. When you said twenty-four, I thought you meant twenty-four thousand. Our minimum is one hundred. Did you know you can order chicks from Sears?" Before I could answer, he went on. "Hey, tell you what, I'll set aside twenty-four for the kid. You can pick them up this afternoon. Just ask for Pete."

When Kevin and I arrived at the hatchery, Pete pretty much ignored me, instead focusing on laying out all the dos and don'ts for raising chickens to Kevin. Once the chicks were boxed up and ready to go, I asked Pete how much we owed him.

"For Kevin, they're free. Besides, the time spent doing the paperwork would cost me more than it's worth."

Those chickens were super layers. Kevin got between eleven and twelve dozen extra-large, often double-yolk brown eggs per week. He sold them for a dollar a dozen and had people lining up to buy them even though eggs were cheaper in the stores.

For myself, meanwhile, I built a fifty-by-seventy-five-foot vegetable garden, which the deer promptly destroyed. For Bonnie, I built four hutches for the rabbits. "Don't put the male bunny in with the females," I told her, "unless you're willing to sell the baby rabbits."

But Bonnie loved those babies, even if she got to play with them for only a little while. With every new litter, we posted an ad in the papers, explicitly designating the rabbits as pets. The same guy came every time and bought every single one. I didn't have the heart to tell her what he was probably doing with them.

LITTLE BOY LOST

On May 3, 1968, the Clark Elementary School bus stopped along Tiger Mountain Road. Eight-year-old David Adams and my son Kevin got off and headed to David's house to ask his mother, Ann, if he could come over to play. David wanted to see the animals on our little farm. She gave her permission, and they headed out, cutting through the property that backed up against David's home to get to the dirt road that led to ours. At five o'clock, David called his mother to see if he could stay longer, but she told him no because it was dinnertime. Kevin walked with David down a trail that led to the bridge crossing Fifteenmile Creek. Because this was the first time David had been to our house, Kevin asked if he wanted him to show him where to cut through to get to his house. David told Kevin that he knew how to get home from there.

The bridge was about ninety feet below grade, so David was out of Kevin's line of sight by the time he reached the top. Fifteen minutes later, the phone rang. Joyce was fixing dinner; I picked up. It was Ann, calling to ask to talk to her son.

"He should be home by now," I said. "He left right after he called you."

There was a pause. "He's not here yet."

"I'll be right there. I'll see if he got lost."

This is where things got confusing. No one knew what path David had taken once he crossed the bridge and got to the top of the hill on the other side. Did he cut through the property, as he and Kevin had coming to our place, or did he go to Tiger Mountain Road and walk around to his street? To our knowledge, the last person to see him was Kevin.

By the time I got to the Adams' house, Ann had called the police. I waited with her for the King County detective sheriff to arrive. He had called the German Shepherd Search Dogs in, and when they got there, the top handler approached me for information about the area and then asked if I would go along with one of the dog handlers, a tall, wiry woman with legs that were at least ten inches longer than mine. We were assigned a heavily wooded and hilly area, and I showed her around, one of her steps equaling one and a half of mine. Later I found out that another dog led his handler to the home of a twenty-year-old Vietnam vet who later became a person of interest. But that all-night search did not find David.

The disappearance of an eight-year-old made news in the *Seattle Post-Intelligencer*, the *Seattle Times*, the *Issaquah Press*, and on local radio and television. This "news" was full of speculation, and it was obvious that most of the reporters didn't know anything about the area, or maybe about woods in general. Theories included David falling down a mine shaft; sinking in quicksand; and being attacked by a cougar, a pack of coyotes, or a bear, then dragged off and eaten. Our house was in a wooded area, but the likelihood of any of these events coming to pass was small if not nil. There were abandoned coal mines in the region, but they were at least a mile east of our house, at the base of Tiger Mountain, and a body eaten by animals would have been easy for the dogs to trace. Anyway, my theory, and the one accepted by officials, was that either David had cut through the property that backed up to his parents' backyard, or he had walked down a road that dead-ended at Tiger Mountain Road, then walked west another four hundred feet to the road he lived on.

Because of the news, people started showing up to "help" search for David. The deluge came when Jim French, a talk radio host on KIRO, announced that more searchers were needed the next day. He was a friend of the family and only trying to help, but more than one thousand searchers showed up that Saturday and quickly covered any vestige of David's scent, making the use of search dogs pointless. From then on, well-intentioned but unequipped folks on foot, bicycle, and horseback roamed the area.

David's dad, Don, was a captain and pilot in the air force reserve, and he'd been called to active duty in Oklahoma because of the USS *Pueblo* incident, when North Korea seized a US Navy surveillance ship three months earlier, in late January of 1968. The air force sent helicopters with a secret infrared system—a new invention at the time—to fly over the area during the second night. That same day, a small group showed up at our house with sledgehammers and crowbars, determined to rip up our flooring to look for David underneath. They left, without apologizing, when they found out that the floor was a slab of concrete. It had truly turned into a circus—a local store had even loaned a refrigerated truck to store food for the searchers. All that was needed was a little car packed with twenty-five clowns to show up.

The police finally called off the search after a week. Despite one of the dogs going to the twenty-year-old vet's house, the police didn't suspect foul play. That year of 1968, in a place where people knew their neighbors and rarely locked their doors, was more than a decade before the "stranger danger" panic. In 2009, the King County Sheriff's Office investigators received a $500,000 grant to reexamine cold cases, and in their new work on the case, they revisited the neighbor's involvement. By that time, he was in his early sixties and living in Eastern Washington, and there was no evidence to tie him to the case. It was as though David had simply vanished into thin air. For as long as I live, I will wonder what happened to him, and regret my not being there to walk him home.

FOLLOW THE SCENT

The week after the search, a car appeared in our driveway. I watched from the window as it came to a stop and two people got out. I recognized them as members of the German Shepherd Search Dogs group and went out to meet them.

"Hello," I said, walking toward them with my hand out to shake. "What can I do for you?"

"We were impressed with the way you worked with the group last week," said the woman who had been my partner in the search, shaking my hand. "Have you considered joining the GSSD?"

"Huh," I said, glancing up toward the house. "I appreciate that, but there's a slight problem."

"Oh yeah?"

"Yeah. Our miniature poodle."

"How do you think your poodle will feel about getting a friend?"

The following week, they delivered Black Bart, a German shepherd with a mainly black coat, thus his name, and some light tan down his chest and lower legs and around his eyes and nose. He was approximately one year old. "A gift for you, since he has little chance of becoming a champion because of his coloring," my former search partner told me. "It's best to train them before they are fully grown, which is eighteen months for this breed."

Joyce fell in love with Bart, so they brought a second puppy, an eight-month-old named Baron Manfred Freiherr von Richthofen IV. While Baron had perfect coloring, his shape would have disqualified him. He and Joyce bonded immediately and became inseparable.

We did not use treats to train the dogs. Their reward was us being pleased. This worked well, even as the training got more difficult. To start, one of my kids, usually Kevin, hid nearby, and I would give the command "FIND," then release Bart and kind of lead him to the "lost" person. Unlike bloodhounds, who are on leash and follow the scent left on the ground, German shepherds work off leash and pick up the scent in the air. When he found the person, I would make a big fuss, telling him what a great dog he was, scratching behind his ears, anything to show him how happy I was. I did make one big mistake, however. Do you know how many times a person says "find" in a day? *I can't find the Phillips screwdriver. Find out what time they want you there. Will you help me find my glasses?* Every time I used the word, which was often, Bart would head to the door. When I heard another handler tell his dog "GO SEEK," a lightbulb lit up above my head. *Darn*, I thought. But it was too late to change commands.

As the training advanced, the designated "lost" person hid farther away. Then they hid in the hollow of a cedar tree stump, or up in a tree, in the brush, or just kept on moving. Sometimes I had Bart search when there was no one around. I saved my jubilation and celebration for when he found someone; however, he did get praised for going on a search even if it were unsuccessful. To up the ante, friends and then people Bart had never met replaced family members, and the German Shepherd Search Dogs held training sessions, sometimes far afield in the wilderness of the Cascades. The King County Sheriff's Office search division held weekend search mockups, which included the German Shepherd Search Dogs, an Explorer Scout search troop, Four-by-Four search group, the Mountaineers, and the Civil Air Patrol. We would set out to find "lost" and "injured" people who'd been planted in the woods to be rescued.

Hope for finding David Adams waned while Bart got better at his job, and I signed us up to be on call twenty-four seven for searches for lost children. This was long before cell phones, so I had a phone line installed in the cabin, and when we finally moved into the big house, a rotary phone stayed on my nightstand so the sheriff could reach me in the middle of the night—search dogs and their trainers need to be the first responders so that the scent of the lost person hasn't yet mixed with other people's scents. I kept my search gear in a special closet, and whenever I got it out, Bart would head straight for the door without me having to say the magic word. I must have emitted some emotion that my dog could sense, because whenever the sheriff's deputy called about a search, Bart would get ready.

SEEK AND YE SHALL FIND

One spring evening, the phone rang. It was after dark and so I assumed that it was the sheriff. This one was a search for two thirteen-year-old girls who were having a sleepover and had not returned from a walk in the woods. They had been gone for three hours.

Several handlers were assigned areas to search. Bart and I had been out for about an hour when we came across a railroad trestle bridge. I stopped and sat on one of the ties to take a drink of water and rest a little. As I was sitting there, I saw a set of headlights coming down a logging road toward the footbridge over the creek below. I took out my binoculars and watched as two young girls got out of a light-blue Ford pickup. I stood up. "I believe I've found the persons," I said into my citizen-band two-way radio. "Code one, over." That meant "alive and well." Anyone could listen in on these radios—it was rare that our chatter was not picked up by non-search people—and we kept our communication vague because we did not want the public to know anything before the deputy sheriff and next of kin.

Bart and I met the girls at the bridge. "My search dog and I were called in by the sheriff," I told them. "You've got some people really worried."

The girls looked at each other. "Please," said one of them. "Please, don't tell my parents. My dad will kill me."

"I report to the deputy, not to you or your parents," I replied. "I'll have to tell the deputy sheriff that you got out of a light-blue Ford pickup truck, including the license number and location. I'll also have to tell him that the truck was occupied by two young males. What he does with that information is up to him."

We had a number of calls to search for missing kids at Rainier School, a center for individuals with intellectual and developmental disabilities located in Buckley, in Pierce County. The property paralleled White River, which was the boundary between King and Pierce Counties, with forest to the east. The school had no restrictive structures, so residents periodically wandered off. As a rule, the kids were easy to find—often they used nearby fields for, well, the usual thing kids sneak off to do. Once, however, we arrived at about ten p.m., and a little after midnight, the search was called off because the missing boy's mother, who lived ten miles from the school in Bonney Lake, heard a knock at the door. When she opened it, there stood her son.

Then there were the mushroom hunters. People who hunt for wild mushrooms, I learned, tend to look at the ground and don't always watch where they're going. One trio of women—a daughter, mother, and grandmother—got lost not once but twice. On their second annual wild mushroom foraging adventure, I heard the grandmother, Gertie, say, "I told you the dogs would find us," when Bart and I showed up.

"We got to—no, we *are going to* stop meeting this way," I said.

"I'm cold," Gertie said, ignoring my statement. Shaking my head, I gave her my down coat. She put it on, then pointed at two five-gallon plastic buckets filled with mushrooms. "You mind carrying those back?"

When we got back to the base, Gertie's husband told her that the only place she was going to hunt for mushrooms was in the produce section of the grocery store. The next day, I asked the deputy if he could see about getting my coat back. He called to let me know that she claimed I'd never loaned her a coat.

One search, in particular, stands out in my memory. It was late on a summer's night, and it had been raining for a couple of days. A three-year-old girl had been gone for hours, and we feared the worst. I'd packed my down sleeping bag, in case I found her and she had hypothermia—rescue blankets would not be available for two more years. As the sun started to rise, turning the sky from black to violet, Bart and I entered a small meadow. On the far side was what looked like a pond; Bart took off in a run. I saw where he was headed, and my heart filled with sorrow. There, lying facedown at the edge of the pool, was the little girl. After whatever had happened to David Adams, I just couldn't bear the thought of facing another grieving parent.

When I got there, however, she moved—I guess she'd thought the little rain-soaked spot was the perfect place for a rest, and she had been asleep with her head on her arm. Adrenaline shot through me as I realized she was OK. I got her into the sleeping bag, which was twice her size, and on an adrenaline high, I carried her all the way back. When I called in the code that she was found and alive, I could hear cheering in the background.

Not all searches were so successful. One summer morning, Bart and I were called out to search for a man in his nineties who lived alone. His wife had died a decade earlier, and he was known for picking wild blackberries. Not just any blackberries; he would pick the trailing blackberry (*Rubus ursinus*), the only blackberry native to Washington. These are smaller than the invasive Himalayan blackberry and have fewer berries, and the taste is superior by far. They are not easy to find. The old man knew a prime spot northeast of Mount Vernon, and every year, he would harvest two bucketsful, make blackberry jam, and give it as thank-you gifts to his friends and neighbors who loved and watched out for him.

It was a quick and easy find. From base, Bart went straight to him. The man was sitting under a tree, leaning back against the trunk. I approached, thinking he was asleep. He had a serene look on his face, and he was still. Too still. He had died doing the thing he loved.

ALL HELL BROKE LOOSE

When I wasn't with my family or going on searches with Bart, I was working hard at my job at Seattle Community College. Things were changing and fast, and the year of 1969 began with a bang in the form of the inauguration of Richard Milhous Nixon. The two-year Summer of Love was still in full swing. In July, Neil Armstrong would walk on the moon, and the following month, more than four hundred thousand people would attend Woodstock in Bethel, New York. All over the country, people were protesting to end war and to win equal rights for marginalized Americans. John Lennon and Yoko Ono staged a week-long bed-in to spread the word about giving peace a chance. Patrons of underground gay bar Stonewall Inn rioted after a police raid. The National Organization for Women demonstrated at the White House with the slogan "Rights, not roses." Thousands of people marched against the Vietnam War, and clashes broke out on campuses across the country as Black students fought for equal rights and access to education.

In terms of political and social unrest, SCC was no exception. The neighborhoods of Capitol Hill and the nearby Central District were a cultural mosaic, a place where people of all races and backgrounds lived and worked side by side. In 1965, the population of the area was nearly 75 percent Black, and the following year, Edison Technical School, a vocational school that had opened in 1921 and that operated out of various school buildings in the area, became part of SCC.

In 1969, $33 million was set to fund SCC and launch two more colleges, one in South Seattle and one in North Seattle. But only $2 million was earmarked for SCC, which just so happened to have a majority Black student population and a vocational focus, while the other two colleges, located in primarily white neighborhoods and designed to be the pathway to four-year degrees, got the lion's share of the funding. Not only that, but there was not a single person of color on the SCC board.

Notice any racial disparity? The people living in the Central District certainly did.

For three weeks in May 1969, the Black Student Union (BSU) led a student strike. The college occupied eleven different sites, and we got bomb threats almost daily at different buildings. A bomb went off at the door of the furnace room of the Summit building—it was loud but fortunately did little damage.

To protest the use of white-only contractor labor in construction on campus, Black contractors formed the Central Contractors Association. Word got out that they were going to storm the construction site, so white workers fortified the site with large boards and bricks to drop on them. From my office, I saw a group of several hundred protesters gather in the park just east of the college, then cut across Broadway and head north in the direction of the construction. The riot police left the entrance to the Broadway High building that they were protecting and rushed to cut them off. Just as the protestors marched past the front entrance, however, they changed course and entered the Broadway High building, first running to the library, where several protestors broke off table legs to use as clubs to break the windows out of all the doors. I met them at the fifth-floor science department—the south wing housed very expensive science equipment that I had worked hard to procure and could not bear to see destroyed. I was standing there, shaking in my shoes and trying to look tough, and they were looking around as if they didn't know where to go; I pointed to the other end of the hall and, in a normal voice, said, "The exit stairs are that way." I was dumbfounded when they turned and left.

The BSU continued to rally with the backing of Students for a Democratic Society. Much as in the protests of Black Lives Matter in Capitol Hill in 2020, there were those who attempted to keep the protests peaceful and those who did not. And, of course, the police did not always do their best to de-escalate, and often resorted to unnecessary force. Violence erupted at Garfield High School, with tear gas and gunshots. Nine police were injured and thirty rioters were arrested.

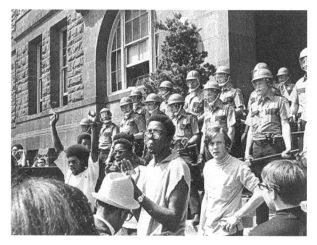

Robert Davis, Jr., leading protest, Seattle Central College, May 22, 1969

BSU demanded that every one of the five all-white board of trustees resign and five Black people be appointed in their place. Instead, one of the trustees resigned, but Governor Dan Evans refused to appoint anyone that the BSU recommended. After two of his picks declined the offer, the governor finally managed to appoint Marvin E. Glass, a Black engineer and supervisor for Pacific Northwest Bell, in July.

Ultimately, Seattle Central joined the other colleges in offering affordable classes that could be part of a four-year degree. To this day, people of color and allies continue the tradition of fighting for equality in Seattle.

AN EARLY RETIREMENT

Though I respected the student protestors' position—attempted destruction of expensive science equipment notwithstanding—I savored my time out in nature, away from the necessary struggle for change. On off days, I would take Bart out into the woods to walk and just be quiet.

Bart loved to search so much that it was his downfall. After three and a half years on the job, Bart picked up the scent of the missing person on a big cedar stump and headed straight for it. There was a window frame and glass leaning against the stump, and I watched in horror as Bart attempted a leap but didn't quite make it to the top. His front right leg broke through the glass, which severed the ligaments of his paw.

The veterinarian told me that he could not do much to save the use of that paw, but that he would try. I left Bart overnight, and when I came back the next day, the vet said he'd contacted one of his graduate professors at the College of Veterinarian Medicine at Washington State University. "They've been doing experimental work with Teflon, using it as a grafting material in surgical interventions," he told me. "If Bart doesn't mind being a guinea pig, they would be happy to see if they could save the use of his paw."

After the operation, the vet warned me not to let Bart do anything that might strain his foot. Which meant no searching for a month. The second week into his recovery, I got a call for a search. As usual, Bart went to the front door to wait for me. I knew that if I opened the door, he would dart out, so I put him out on the top back deck and asked Joyce to let him back in after I'd gone. When I closed the front door, however, he jumped over the railing and dropped twenty-plus feet to the ground, landing on his paws and tearing the Teflon loose. The next day, I called the veterinarian college at WSU, but that mad leap was the final straw. The paw was unrepairable.

AN ENDING

In the summer of 1971, I worked on a project, granted by the National Science Foundation, to develop a new two-year associate of science chemistry technician degree program for community colleges. I was writing textbooks and laboratory manuals with a group of college and university professors at the University of California, Berkeley. I got home just in time to surprise Vicki for her birthday in August. She saw me driving up and met me at the door with a big hug. Then Joyce came up behind her and said, "I want you to leave."

That was the final straw on what had been a long, slow pileup of dysfunction in our marriage. We'd been together going on seventeen years, and for most of that time, Joyce had been unhappy. I tried to follow my dad's advice and create romance however I could, but nothing worked. In the last few years, whenever I asked her to go on a date, she found a reason not to go. This eventually became, simply, "I don't want to go." The last time I brought her flowers, she put them down the garbage disposal. In all those years, we'd had friends over to the house just three times; she only spoke when directly spoken to and nothing more. I don't remember being invited to anyone's house other than our parents'. I'd given her an ultimatum: we needed to do something, anything, within a year, or else I wanted a divorce. A year came and went. I moved out, back into the little cabin we'd all shared when the house was being built.

I'm sure that if you asked Joyce, she'd have a different version of events. But this is my book.

Shortly thereafter, I moved into an apartment in Capitol Hill, ten blocks from the college. The apartment did not allow pets, and Joyce did not want Bart because she had Baron. The vet helped me find someone to adopt him, a man in his eighties who used a wheelchair because his right leg had been amputated above the knee and he was in need of an emotional support dog (though we didn't use that designation at the time). I was cautioned not to visit while Bart and his new owner were bonding, and I heard that it was a great match. Like so many relationships in my life, I didn't have too much trouble letting go.

Our divorce was finalized at the end of 1972. We sold the house for twice what it cost to build. Joyce bought a new place in Issaquah so that the kids could continue with their schooling there.

We'd married too young. Now we were grown. A new phase had begun.

CHAPTER 11

Bachelorhood

I loaded up my little two-door Honda 600 with my belongings and headed to Capitol Hill. My new apartment building on Melrose Avenue faced the I-5 freeway, and my one-bedroom apartment was on the top floor. It didn't take me long to get settled in. Every morning, I walked to work at Seattle Central College, and when I got home in the evenings, I would put a twelve-inch vinyl record on the turntable, usually instrumental soft jazz or classical, turn off the lights, sit in my favorite chair, and chill out. I kept the deck's sliding door closed to block out the freeway noise, which gave me a glass wall with an unbelievable panoramic view. To the south were the ferry docks and the Seattle waterfront; straight ahead were the lights of downtown and the Space Needle, the Puget Sound, and Bainbridge Island with a backdrop of the Olympic Mountains. To the north, the giant Queen Anne Hill rose into the sky. The seaplanes flew due east, straight toward my apartment, then turned at a right angle to land on Lake Union. At night, their landing lights would suddenly sweep my apartment, surprising more than one guest caught in the glare.

I had never lived alone. The kids were with Joyce in Issaquah so they could stay in their schools. Vicki would be graduating from Issaquah High School in June; Bonnie was a sophomore, and Scott, Susan, and Kevin were in middle school. I saw them on weekends, taking them to plays and concerts and other standard divorced-dad activities. When the younger kids were in high school, I bought them a 1966 Mercury Monterey Breezeway four-door sedan so they could come out and see me. Susan loved to drive, and I got the impression that she had control of the keys and spent most of her time wearing out the tires with friends.

After being married for seventeen years, I'd thought bachelorhood was going to feel strange, and that it would be awkward trying to get back into dating. But it was a whole new world out there, and I was a different person. I was neither young nor religious, and I didn't really think my sex life was anybody's business, not even God's. On top of that, it was the 1970s. Second-wave feminism was in full effect, with activists fighting for equal opportunity and equal pay for equal work. Betty Friedan's *The Feminine Mystique* had almost a decade under its belt. Gloria Steinem was everywhere, and Kate Millett's book *Sexual Politics* had just come out. New laws and the *Roe v. Wade* ruling in 1973 gave women more reproductive freedom and access to birth control. That same year, ninety million people watched tennis champ Billie Jean King wipe the court with Bobby Riggs in their world-famous Battle of the Sexes, bolstering support for Title IX. Women even won the right to have their own credit cards and apply for their own mortgages! (For younger people, the fact that women didn't always have those basic financial freedoms might sound outrageous, but it's true.) Suddenly, no-fault divorces like mine were common.

These incredible changes brought about a big change in dating. Way back when, in my LDS community in the 1950s, the expectation was that you dated one person exclusively with a goal of marriage, and if you determined matrimony was not in the cards, then you broke up. Sex was reserved for after you and your bride said "I do" and signed the paperwork. This was no longer in vogue. Many people dated casually and had open or nonexclusive relationships. It was even acceptable for women to ask men out, which for me came as a happy surprise.

A couple weeks after I'd moved into my new apartment, my friend Tom told me about a singles group bowling night that Saturday. "You should come," he said.

"I don't know—"

"C'mon, it'll be fun. There are always more women than men. You should drive because the gals tend to carpool, and if you meet someone you like, you can offer her a ride home. That," he added, "is how I met my new girlfriend. Either way, it's just bowling."

That didn't sound too bad. That Saturday, I arrived to find a group of folks mostly in their thirties and forties hanging around and putting on bowling shoes. "Hey, everyone," Tom yelled out. "I want you to meet my friend Herb. This is his first time with the group, so make him feel welcome—especially you gals without a partner."

A woman with short brown hair, glasses, and tight bell-bottom jeans pushed her way through, reaching out her hand to shake. "Hi," she said. "I'm Paulette. Welcome to my team, team number three. I've got you down to bowl right after me. That will give us time to get better acquainted."

By the end of the first game, I had asked Paulette if she wanted a ride home. "I just need to tell Denise that I won't be riding with her," she said. Later I found out that Paulette was the driver and actually needed to give her car keys to her friend. At the end of the evening, Joella, another woman on our team, approached me as I was bent over, taking off my bowling shoes. With a wink and a smile, she slipped a note in my shirt pocket. *I cook a mean dinner. If you're interested, let me know. xo Joella.* After her name was her phone number.

What an icebreaker that evening was. After a couple of months of dating, Paulette started talking more and more about what a great husband and father I would be for her two daughters and son. I was definitely not ready to get married again, and my five kids were more than enough. Besides, Joella did, in fact, cook a mean dinner.

Over time, I would realize that I had to make my intentions clear up front. I was not looking for a wife, and I was already a father. When the hints at commitment started, I would withdraw with as much respect and honesty as possible. I didn't want back on that merry-go-round.

I also came up with a few rules, mostly by trial and error. No married women. No one who worked for me or worked above me. No students. One result of all those new no-fault divorces was that Seattle Central College's typical student was a thirty-two-year-old divorced woman with two kids working on a degree to get a job to support her family. My Chemistry 101 class just so happened to be a prerequisite for aspiring nurses, and more than once, I had to turn down a date with someone whom I might've said yes to if we'd met in another setting.

And finally: no women who lived in my apartment building. I added this rule after observing the potential fallout if things were to go awry. One evening, I knocked on the door of that night's date, and the door across the hall cracked open and a man peeked out. "Hi!" I said. He slammed the door. I didn't think much of it until I was in my date's apartment and there was a knock on her door. When she opened it, there stood Peekaboo Man.

"You got some Scotch tape I can borrow?" he said, giving me the once-over.

"Fine," she said, rifling through a drawer and then handing him the roll with a glare.

Once he'd left, I said, "That's different than the old adage about borrowing a cup of sugar."

"I dated him for a while. This is his little routine. He'll bring it back in thirty minutes."

It was twenty.

At the end of the night, we were saying our goodbyes in the doorway when the ex's door creaked open. "I had a wonderful time," I said. Then, to get his goat, I leaned in and planted a big kiss on her, which she enthusiastically returned. After a moment, I heard a throat being cleared across the hall. She broke away, smiled, and said a final good night before closing her door. As I left, I gave him a thumbs-up. "It was a great evening!" I said with a wink.

DON'T JUDGE A CHEM PROF BY HIS JOB TITLE

One Saturday afternoon, I was perusing the albums at 65th Street Records in Ravenna when a poster in the window caught my eye. It was an ad for Seattle Gilbert & Sullivan Society's double feature *Sorcerer* and *Trial by Jury*, which brought back memories of my own stint in a Gilbert & Sullivan production in high school. At the checkout counter, the clerk and I got to talking, and Mary told me that she was the second lead female in *Sorcerer.* "Oh really?" I said. "I built sets in high school for a Gilbert and Sullivan show."

She put my purchase down on the counter. "Would you be interested in helping us out?"

Mary gave me the name of the artistic director and location, and when I arrived the following weekend, introduced myself to Gordon Gutteridge, and told him that Mary had said he could use my help, his body language clearly conveyed, *The hell I do,* while he said, "I might be able to find something you could work on." He handed me a sheet of paper listing the dimensions of five shipping-box props, and after asking a few questions about their appearance and purpose, I strapped on my tool belt and headed to the wood stack.

In less than an hour, I called out to Gordon, "Do you want me to use muslin on the sides to keep the weight down? If so, where's the muslin and glue?"

Gordon walked over to check my work. "I can't believe you've gotten this far," he said after a couple minutes. "How did you do it so quickly?"

"I've worked with wood since I was old enough to use a hammer and know which end of a nail to hit," I told him. "I helped my dad, uncle, and grandfather build their houses, and I built my family's three-story house a year and a half ago. And I was in charge of building sets and props and staging for my school's productions my junior year of high school."

He stood up and hooked his thumbs through the belt loops on his jeans. "When you said you were a chemistry prof, I thought you would just get in my way. I owe you an apology." I nodded. "All right, then. The muslin and glue are on the shelves back by the wood. When you finish with the muslin, you can help me build flats."

That was the beginning of a long and close friendship. I also made friends with cast and orchestra members. And, yes, there were several single women.

Seattle Gilbert & Sullivan Society did only one two-week production per year. The orchestra and much of the cast also performed for Sound Expression Theater (SET), located in Edmonds; they did four two-week productions a year. Ellen Lund, the concertmaster and president of SET, asked me to help build sets, assist the gaffer (lighting technician), and stage-manage the shows. I did so mainly so that I could have my sons work with me. Scott worked the first season before graduating from high school and getting a job as a computer programmer. Kevin continued working in theater until he retired.

SET had hired professionals for the roles of artistic director/director, music director, set designer, and costume designer. Their combined salaries added up to more than ticket sales for a season, and SET ended up closing. The artistic director, Ron Daum, called me after the dust had settled to talk about starting a new theater group. He had moved to Seattle from Hollywood and fallen in love with the Northwest, and he wanted to stay. Marni Nixon, "ghost singer" for Audrey Hepburn; Natalie Wood; and Deborah Kerr, the singing nun in *The Sound of Music*, were also at the meeting that formed MusiComedy Northwest theater group. We eventually found a home at Seattle Repertory Theatre's Second Stage. I ended up being producer, set designer and builder, and technical director for the first year, using Marni Nixon's garage for my set shop. This turned into a few invitations to dinner.

By this time, Kevin had gained enough skill and know-how through working alongside his dear ol' dad and taking a summer class in set building that we hired him as technical director and light designer. He was fifteen going on sixteen and a hard worker, and it was a job he could do while still in high school. It was interesting to watch union stagehands learn to take orders from him—it took a minute, but quickly they realized that he knew what he was doing. Besides, I was close by if he needed me.

RULES ARE MADE TO BE BROKEN

In October of 1976, the building manager moved my parking place to a more convenient location, just to the right of the walkway into the building and next to a sage-green Plymouth. I caught glimpses of the woman driving it, but I didn't pay all that much attention. That is, until the evening I pulled up to find that sage-green Plymouth parked in my spot.

The next morning, as I headed down to the sixth-floor exit, I saw a woman crossing the walkway below. I'll just say that the back of her was a pleasing sight, and she had beautiful red hair, the kind you can't get out of a bottle. She got in the Plymouth in my spot and, before I could get a good look at her, drove off. That evening, I just so happened to pull up as this same woman was walking out of the mail room on the walkway-level floor. Curiosity got the better of me, and I watched to see which apartment she entered, then looked her up on the residence roster: G. Kortus. I found her phone number in the phone book and immediately called her.

When she answered, I said, "Hello. Are you the person who owns the sage-green Plymouth that was parked in my spot last night?"

There was a pause. "Yes," she answered after a moment. "I'm sorry I parked in your spot. I got home after dark, and someone was in my spot, and, well, I knew a man had the spot next to mine and it would be safer for him to park on the street than it would be for me."

"Ah," I said. "I see. That was the right thing for you to do. Please feel free to park there in the future if someone is parked in your spot."

We talked for almost an hour, and Gloria accepted my invitation to a dinner date the following evening. Later she told me that she had had a glass of wine with her good friend Janice after work that afternoon, which was why she was so friendly and amenable. *I just accepted a blind date with someone I've never met,* she'd thought. *I must be out of my mind. Or it's the wine.* The next day, she checked the residence roster and called Janice to give her my name, address, and car license number, in case I turned out to be a creep. "If you don't hear from me by midnight," she said, "call the police."

There went Dating Rule Number Four: no woman who lived in my apartment building. But, I reasoned, she lived on the fourth floor at the north end, and I lived on the sixth floor at the south end. If the date went down in flames, we'd be able to avoid each other.

When Gloria opened her door, I was pleasantly surprised. Standing in front of me was a woman of understated beauty, one of those rare people who don't need makeup, jewelry, or elaborate clothing to look pretty. She was wearing a pale-pink pleated blouse with a burgundy skirt and oxblood flats, nude lipstick, and a little gold teddy bear pendant with a diamond-chip belly button on a short gold chain.

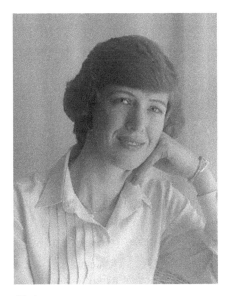

Gloria

As we walked to my car, Gloria kept space between us, and once inside, she leaned up against the passenger-side door, both hands resting on her right leg. Her body language said, *You're probably not Jack the Ripper, but I'll stay right over here just in case.*

During dinner, she relaxed as our conversation flowed. Our phone call of the previous evening had established the basics, and now I found out more. She had grown up on a farm in Whatcom County, the firstborn, who, by not being a boy, had disappointed her father from day one. Theirs was a deeply religious family that attended a very conservative evangelical church—she did not go to prom, and she didn't see a movie until she was eighteen. Farm chores came before schoolwork, and often she had to do her homework under the blanket by flashlight. Even so, she'd graduated salutatorian, but her parents didn't support her choice to leave home to attend ITT Peterson School of Business. Now she worked for Wards Cove Packing, a job that took her to Alaska for five months every year. "I don't plan on getting married," she told me, "or having kids. I like my work, and I like the freedom to come and go as I please."

"I've been married," I said, "and I don't plan on getting married again. And I've already done my share of being fruitful and multiplying."

Those first hours with Gloria flew by. As we waited for our dessert to arrive, she reached over and took my hand. "I'm glad you called me," she said. "This has been a wonderful night."

I gave her hand a squeeze. "Thank you for parking in my parking spot. It was well worth having to find parking on the street. But just so you know, you don't have to park there again to get me to ask you out on another date."

We spent a few minutes talking outside her front door; all the while, I was thinking, *Should I kiss her good night?* Before I could, she said in a rush, "Sorry, but I have to go," and hurried inside.

The next day, she called me to tell me why she'd exited our date so abruptly. She'd realized it was just before midnight, and if she didn't call Janice soon, the police would come looking for me. We both laughed, then got to figuring out when and where the next date would be. Gloria suggested bowling—little did I know that a row of bowling trophies for season averages greater than 250 lined her bookcase, and that she had a little test for me in mind.

On the way to the bowling alley, she asked, "How would you feel if I outscored you tonight?"

"I'd feel that you are a better bowler than I am."

"Would that bother you?"

"Why should it?"

"Because I'm a woman and you're a man. I once had a boyfriend who broke up with me over bowling."

"If he was that egotistical, you're better off without him. I'm just here to spend time with you and enjoy the evening."

I surprised both of us by winning the first game—truly, I was not trying to prove a point, and I had never done that well in my life, nor would I ever again. Second game, she trounced me. I passed her test—I could not have cared less about being outscored by a woman.

Our third date was a picnic on the lawn at Ballard Locks, and by Christmas, we were basically a couple. We celebrated our first Valentine's Day together in February of 1977, and from then on, Valentine's Day was our biggest holiday, the day we celebrated our love.

Just as she'd warned me, Gloria left for work at the Alitak Cannery on Lazy Bay, at the southern tip of Kodiak Island, Alaska, three months later. The four previous years, whatever boyfriend she had in May exited stage left when they found out she would be gone for five months. I was the first to take her to the airport and pick her up when she returned in September.

For the next six years, we spent seven months together and five months apart every year. A World War II–era eight-passenger Grumman G-21 Goose amphibious airplane delivered my love letters three times a week, as well as a single yellow rosebud from a flower shop in Kodiak. When the florist told me that the delivery charge would be the same for one rose as it was for two dozen, I told her, "One rose says 'I love you' more than two dozen."

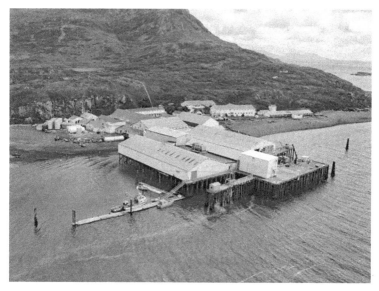

Alitak Cannery

As Lucille Ball once said, "Once in his life, every man is entitled to fall madly in love with a gorgeous redhead."

CHAPTER 12

A Glass of Wine and a Talk

In May of 1979, Gloria was getting ready for her annual summer trip to the Alitak Cannery. We had been together for two and a half years, and this year, instead of spending a few months apart, she wanted me to go with her. "You'll understand why I love it there," she told me. I suspect she wanted to show, rather than tell, why she was determined to keep her job, to keep this part of her life. It was the 1970s, after all, and generally white middle-class women were expected to stay home and settle down once they'd found a man.

I'm always open to a new adventure, and a trip to Alaska with my gorgeous redheaded girlfriend seemed like fun. I knew she'd be working, so I got a construction job building two new bunkhouses.

The cannery was not what I expected. It was in about the most isolated place I'd ever been. The only way to get there was by boat or seaplane. One lonely planted tree towered above the low shrubs, grasses, and mosses of the tundra. The cannery itself would have fit on a football field. The water came through a wooden pipe from a lake on a hill behind it; electricity came via giant generators. There was nothing to do but work, eat, sleep, and play horseshoes in the one horseshoe pit. There was one basketball hoop, too, but I never did see a basketball. The workers had up to sixteen-hour shifts, three regular meals in the mess hall, and three "mug-ups" (coffee and pastry breaks) at nine a.m., three p.m., and nine p.m.

Gloria was a workaholic. She was in the office from before breakfast until the nine p.m. mug-up. I ate my meals in the workers' mess hall, while she ate hers in the administrators' dining room, so we only got to see each other during mug-ups and in the evenings. Sunday was a non-workday for me, and sometimes for Gloria. No one had told me to bring a book, so when she worked on Sundays, I would sneak into the construction site and work—there was nothing else to do.

As hoped, I came to understand why Gloria liked working there so much. On the family farm, she never got a thank-you; instead, she got only grumbles about doing whatever faster or better or more. She could never do anything right in the eyes of her parents, but at Alitak, she was respected, praised, and rewarded. At the cannery, she felt good about herself.

Winn Brindle, her boss, relied heavily on her. She was the go-to person and second in charge, the first female office manager in the company. Apparently, Winn feared that if we got married, I would not want her to leave every summer, and then we'd have children, and then he'd lose her. So he'd started buzzing in her ear. "He's older than you," he told her (and which she later reported to me). "He probably just wants a bunch of kids." Winn went out of his way to keep us apart, never inviting me to the administrators' dining room, and even threatening to send me off to work on a fishing boat.

In most ways, Gloria appreciated her boss's mentorship, and the fact that he treated her like family. But in this way, he was wrong and in need of correction. So Gloria and I scheduled a private mug-up with him in the office. Gloria started the conversation. "Just so you know," she said, "I plan on working summers at Wards Cove as long as you'll have me." He cocked an eyebrow. "And I don't want children," she added.

A look of disbelief crossed his face, so I decided to back up the "no children" promise. "I've had a vasectomy," I told him.

He blanched. This was long before the invention of the phrase "TMI," but he was probably thinking something along those lines. "What the hell did you do that for?" he said after a moment.

"I already have five kids," I said. I also let him know that I liked my summers free, that I took graduate classes and taught at United States and international colleges and universities as a visiting professor.

Winn seemed reassured. On Friday, he told Gloria he was going to take his small floatplane to pick up something in Kodiak, then stay the night and fly back on Saturday afternoon. When he returned, he handed Gloria an envelope and said, "You and Herb get a bag packed. Starting Monday, you two are on vacation for the week. I've made arrangements for you to fly out on the Goose when they bring the mail. There are two round-trip plane tickets to Anchorage, and reservations for a car and a room at the Historic Anchorage Hotel. The American Express card is to cover expenses. Have a great time." Though he never did apologize, this was good enough, an olive branch and a gesture of acceptance. Winn was like an old marshmallow, crusty on the outside but soft in the middle.

A GROUNDBREAKING CONVERSATION

For the Fourth of July, Gloria suggested that we drive out to another Wards Cove processing plant on the Kenai Peninsula.

I was game—this was my first time in Alaska, and I wanted to see as much of it as I could.

We were cruising along Highway 1 when the traffic slowed to a stop at a sign that said, "BLASTING ZONE AHEAD." In front of us, the driver got out of his pickup, threw a blanket on the hood, and laid back on the windshield with a book. Gloria and I looked at each other. "I guess we're in for a long wait," I said.

Our conversation led to Gloria talking about how she always spent Thanksgiving weekend with her aunt Jody and uncle Gene, who lived in Lakewood, California. She asked if I would like to go with her this year.

"Sure!" I said.

"Oh good," Gloria said. "We can go to Disneyland, Knott's Berry Farm, Universal Studios. Maybe visit LA or go to the beach in San Diego."

"You know, I lived in Compton my senior year of high school. It's less than ten miles from Lakewood. I'll have to visit my mom and dad. If Mom ever found out that I was in Southern California and didn't stop by, I'd never hear the end of it. They now live in Lucerne Valley, a couple of hours away."

"I'd love to meet them."

I paused. "Do you realize what we've been talking about?"

"Yeah. Sounds like we're talking about getting married."

"Do you want to?"

"Yes, I would've married you two years ago. Do you want to? I thought you didn't ever want to get married again."

"I love you too much not to. When and where?"

"How about in Seattle, in October when I get home?"

"What about in Paris under the Eiffel Tower?"

"I want to share it with my friends and family."

That pulled me up short. If we were really going to do this, in front of friends and family, I'd need to come clean. "Uh, so . . ." I began, not sure how to phrase what I needed to say. I took a breath. "I told you a little white lie when we first started dating. I, uh, I subtracted five years off my age."

"That's OK," Gloria said. "I added five years to my age."

So much for a romantic dinner by candlelight, with flowers and expensive champagne and kneeling on one knee.

After deciding to get married, we talked about what would make a good marriage. First, we would live off one salary so that the other would be discretionary money. Our salaries were within a couple hundred dollars. I had, by far, the best retirement program, so we would maximize it. We wouldn't spend a thousand or more on an item without discussing it, unless it was a birthday or Christmas present. We would have a shared checking account. When problems arose, we'd discuss them. No yelling, no shouting, no calling names. We'd remember that we'd fallen in love because of who we are, and that love and respect cause change, and that change will bring us closer and make our love deeper. We'd keep our promises. We'd live the golden rule, and we'd have each other's back. Oh yes, one more thing! We'd always say "please" and "thank you."

A few more blasts of dynamite and we were on our way to Kenai. This was a couple decades before GPS, and my copilot missed our turnoff. We continued to the small fishing town of Homer, population five thousand and the Halibut Fishing Capital of the World. A billboard advertised that Homer was also the fun capital of Alaska. They'd had a parade that morning, but everyone must have gone home; the streets were bare, and the ice-cream store only had one flavor left, peppermint. After checking out the town, we passed through Kenai on our way back to Anchorage.

Gloria was excited to call her aunt Jody from the hotel room phone and tell her we were getting married. "There will be an extra person at the Thanksgiving table this year!" she said. After their lengthy conversation, the Anchorage Fourth of July fireworks show started, and we had a prime view out our window. Gloria told her aunt, "Gotta go—Anchorage is celebrating us getting married!"

MEETING THE FAMILIES

When I left Alitak, I remarked to Gloria that I wished I'd brought my camera so I could take a photo of her for my nightstand. She said that she had her photograph taken at a studio for Christmas, and I might be able to get one there. When the clerk informed me that they could not sell one to me without her permission, I explained that she was working in Alaska at a salmon packing plant and there were no phones and communication was by ship-to-shore radio and reserved for emergencies. "Well," she said, "you can get permission from her parents."

I had never met anyone in Gloria's family. I made a cold call from the studio and introduced myself to Gloria's mother, Caroline. "This is Herb Bryce, Gloria's boyfriend," I said.

"I remember her mentioning you," Caroline said. "Why don't you come for dinner Saturday?" It was obvious that Gloria hadn't written her mom to tell her that we were getting married. She did know that we were serious, and even that we were living together, though she told people that Gloria was sleeping on my couch.

Dinner was interesting. Caroline had an appointment in Bellingham that afternoon, so I met her there so I could follow her to the farm. She'd left the chicken on the stove soaking in at least two inches of oil, and put the baked potatoes in the oven that morning so she could just warm them up for dinner. A saucepan with two cans of peas was also waiting to be heated. When we arrived, she turned the burners on high and the oven to 350 degrees.

While dinner was heating, Al, Gloria's dad, invited me to

look around the farm. What he really wanted to do was get things straight about me, Gloria, and the farm. "The Bible says that the oldest son gets fifty percent of the property," he said as we walked along the fence line, "and the other sons split the remainder. Daughters shall not inherit any land. I only have two sons, so they will each get half. If any of my daughters want a farm, they will need to marry a farmer. If you are thinking of marrying Gloria, I want you to know that you and Gloria will not inherit my farm."

The Bible actually says that the firstborn receives a double portion, but it's bad manners to tell the father of your fiancée that he needs to check his Bible. Besides, I don't think that particular edict is fair. "I'm a dean and science teacher at Seattle Central College," I told him, "and I love my job. I'm not interested in your dairy farm."

The meal went fine after that, though the chicken was saturated with oil, the potatoes were dry, and the peas were more like pea soup. I silently thanked God that Gloria hadn't learned how to cook from her mother.

(Many years later, when Gloria's parents were in their midseventies, they deeded the farm to their oldest son because the two brothers refused to work together. In less than a year, he'd sold it. Their old house had a "life estate" agreement, and they wanted to stay there. But the place was a teardown—the roof leaked, it had single-pane windows and no insulation, water stains marred the ceiling and carpets, and worst of all, the well water contained fecal coliform bacteria. Renovations would have cost us more than $100,000 that we would never recoup because the owner would automatically receive the title when they died. My mother said, "You bought me a condo when your dad died, so you need to buy Gloria's parents a place to live." Which we did, on a piece of land about a mile down the road. They lived there until dementia forced them into assisted living, in the first decade of the twenty-first century.)

PLANNING A WEDDING

Without giving a lot of thought to what's involved in planning a wedding, we set the date for October 20, about two weeks after Gloria was set to come home. I returned to Seattle at the beginning of September. For my first wedding twenty-odd years earlier, all I had to do was show up in a suit, with my hair combed and my tie on straight and my shoes polished. I didn't even have to prepare my vows; I just needed to say "I do." This marriage was different for a lot of reasons, including the fact that we, not our parents, were arranging everything. Booking the church was easy because Gloria had been a member for five years. Alcohol was prohibited in the church's recreation hall, so we needed to get a reception hall. Gloria specifically wanted champagne.

That's when reality struck. I called a nearby hotel and asked the hotel manager if I could make a reservation for October 20.

"Eighty or eighty-one?" she asked.

"This October. 1979."

She cleared her throat. "We are booked up for the next year. Two years for the month of June."

I got similar responses from at least a dozen places, but I was determined to get Gloria her champagne. Driving south on I-5 in Lynnwood one afternoon, I noticed a "Grand Opening" banner hanging on the roof of a new hotel. They had a hall available, thank goodness.

Gloria had only ten days to find her bridal outfit; she looked beautiful in an off-the-rack dress with a high lace collar that accentuated the elegant length of her neck and a crown of white daisies that complemented her lovely red hair.

After the simple ceremony, we had hors d'oeuvres, champagne, sparkling apple cider, and cake from a nearby bakery. Friends from the New Deal Rhythm Band played as a gift. All in all, it turned out to be a great wedding. Gloria's friends kept the champagne flowing, and when we got home, Gloria fell asleep in her dress.

Sunday, we headed to Harrison Hot Springs Resort in British Columbia for three nights. We had massages, walked along the shore of Harrison Lake, relaxed in the hot mineral springs pools, ate leisurely meals in the restaurant and the café. On Tuesday morning at three a.m., Gloria said, "Do you want to go skinny-dipping in the heated pool?"

She didn't have to ask me twice. "Let's go," I said.

We put on our robes and tiptoed down to the pool. It was perfect, the steam rising in the darkness. No one was around. We shed our robes at the shallow end and jumped in. We were playing around, doing what newlyweds do, when an elderly man came in, dove into the deep end, and started swimming laps. Thank heavens he didn't turn on the lights. After ten laps, he got out, dried off, and left. Gloria and I put on our robes soaking wet and laughed all the way back to our suite.

SECOND THOUGHTS

As planned, we went to Gloria's aunt Jody's house for Thanksgiving. We flew down on Tuesday and checked into the Hilton Anaheim hotel for one night, planning to walk to Disneyland and play like kids the next day. We had settled in our room when Gloria said, "Let's go down to the lounge and have a glass of wine."

After a couple of sips, Gloria started crying. "I don't want to be married anymore," she said, sniffling. "I work ten to twelve hours a day, then come home and cook dinner and clean the house. I'm tired all the time."

I'd suspected this was coming. When we were happily

living in sin, we'd shared the housework equally. The day after
we got married, she physically pushed me out of the kitchen,
telling me to go sit down and watch the news while she fixed
dinner. If I got out the vacuum, she unplugged it and told me,
again, to go watch the news. Now, I said, "I liked making dinner and cleaning the house before we got married. Why the
big change all of a sudden?"

"I'm your wife now. That's what wives do."

"Do you want to get an annulment and remarry and have
the pastor say, *I now pronounce you friends and partners*?"

"That's silly."

"I know it is. It is just as silly as saying 'I do' and turning
into some kind of farmer's wife. Gloria! I fell in love and married you because of who you are. That person is who I want to
live with for the rest of my life. I don't want you to be 'a wife.'
Just be Gloria!"

She reached across the table, took my hands in hers, and
smiled. "I love you," she whispered. "Thank you."

"I love you, too, and always will."

"Want to finish the wine and go up to our room and be
friends and partners?"

A day of playing like little kids in never-never land was
what we needed, a lighthearted day full of love, fun, and laugh-
ter. On the way to Jody and Gene's, we stopped at Knott's
Berry Farm for Mrs. Knott's famous chicken dinner and deep-
dish boysenberry pie à la mode. That was a mistake—I was still
full on Thanksgiving Day, and Jody cooked enough for a dozen
even though only six were at the table.

On Friday, we headed to Lucerne Valley to visit my parents. Gloria and Mom had fallen in love at our wedding. Now
they were talking as if they'd known each other for years; Dad
and I couldn't get a word in edgewise. At lunch, Dad sat by
Gloria. For a man who didn't say much, especially when my
mom was around, he and Gloria really hit it off, making up for

not having time at our wedding. Sunday night, we returned to Seattle to start our lives as friends and partners and end the farm-wife episode. I fixed breakfast Monday morning.

(I'm glad Dad and Gloria got to spend time together. This would be the last time she saw him. At the end of June the following summer, Gloria was in Alitak when Dad, age seventy-one, had an accident. He was priming the carburetor of an old truck on the farm and had poured gasoline out of a can into the carburetor. Forgetting to step back from the truck, he told his grandson Dennis to try starting the truck. When Dennis turned the key, flames roared out of the carburetor. Dad jumped back, spilling the remaining gas down his front, which caught on fire. Dennis jumped out of the truck, tackled Dad to the ground, and rolled him in the dirt to put out the fire, saving him from third- and fourth-degree external burns. It wasn't until they examined him at the hospital, after a ninety-minute ride in an ambulance, that they found he had fourth-degree burns in his lungs. Mom would not let the hospital "pull the plug" until July 11. Many years later, Mom had a stroke and went into a coma five weeks before her hundredth birthday, and I flew down to see her while Gloria stayed home because it was tax time, and she was CFO. Three days later, Gloria showed up at the hospital. "I had dreams that your mom was waiting for me. I had to come down." She drew up a chair, sat down, and took Mom's hand. "I love you more than words can express," Gloria said. "If it's time for you to go, we understand." Mom died twenty minutes later.)

REAL LIFE

Our real honeymoon was a week-long Caribbean cruise on Norwegian Cruise Lines, in April. The weather was initially stormy, and Gloria was seasick most of the first two days.

Dramamine didn't work, so she went to the infirmary, which offered scopolamine pills in a little plastic bag taped to the door. (That was our first of sixteen cruises, most of which we took with our friends Bill and Jan Schnall. The longest was twenty-nine days, from Hong Kong to Greece. Gloria used the transdermal patch, and seasickness was no longer a problem. We also loved driving, particularly around Europe and the United Kingdom. We visited more than seventy-five countries.)

Gloria could always sense when May was approaching; like a bird, the pull of migration took her to Alitak. While she was there, I taught a summer course of Science for Elementary Teachers through a National Science Foundation grant. This became our annual summertime tradition, with me traveling to various universities to teach teachers. At the University of Northern Colorado, five of us developed a book of thirty-two classroom activities and demonstrations for pre–high school teachers. At Miami University, I helped develop and taught Teaching Science With Toys for elementary teachers. At the University of Puget Sound and Seattle Central College, I taught How to Do Demonstrations for High School and College Teachers, and I used NSF grants to develop science summer camps for minority sixth-grade girls.

During the regular school year, I did workshops and lectures on demonstration at the National Science Teaching Association national conferences. A $10,000 grant bought the supplies and chemicals for demonstrations for schools and at least one big show a year for the public. Most of the big shows were with Tim Hoyt, a chemistry professor at the University of Puget Sound. Tim had long white hair and a big white beard, and he would dress up in a wizard robe and hat, while I donned the classic white science lab coat. We would explain the difference between "magic" and "science": If you don't know why or what made it happen, then it's *magic*. If you know why or what made it happen, then it's *science*.

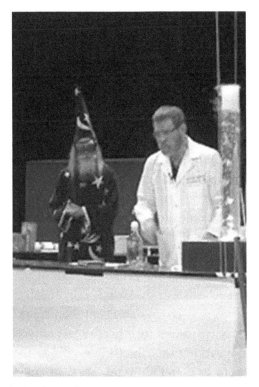

A big show with Tim Hoyt

I was highly active in the national and Puget Sound sections of the American Chemical Society, serving a term as president and representative at the national meetings and on national committees for twelve years. My passion was to help kids understand, participate in, and enjoy science.

The last two summers that Gloria worked in Alitak, I was invited by the Taiwan Ministry of Education to teach chemistry for college instructors. Before I went the first year, they called me to say that I was actually going to teach industrial safety. I assured them that my degree was chemistry, not industrial safety.

"Yes, we know," was the answer, "but you will teach industrial safety." Of the nine American teachers, I was the only academic professor, while the rest were different types of industrial technology instructors.

I called our director and told her what happened, and she told me that the colleges had canceled chemistry technology and, yes, I was going to teach industrial safety. "You better head to the library and bone up on industrial safety," she told me.

When I got to Taiwan, I found out that they did not know the first thing about industrial safety. Welders rode motorbikes with acetylene and oxygen tanks bungee strapped to the back fender through the crowded streets of Taipei. At the government-controlled China Shipbuilding Corporation, an ironworker in shorts and flip-flops, and without a shirt, hard hat, or safety goggles, was using a grinder that was nothing but a motor and two grinding wheels. For the switch, they stripped the installation off the ends of two wires and bent them in a U shape and just hooked the two wires together. The worst was the white-collar workers parking their motorbikes inside the liquid oxygen cage. I had more than four pages' worth of safety violations at the end of the day.

The Ministry of Education insisted I return the next summer, and I was surprised to find that most of the major things I had reported were corrected. I couldn't take full credit—there'd been an explosion at China Steel before my second visit. After that, both factories required safe clothing, hard hats, steel-toed shoes, and safety goggles. No motorbikes in the liquid oxygen cage. Brand-new grinders with a guarded switch. Secured gas tanks with caps.

Two weeks before I was to go home, the organizers asked me to take a leave of absence and move to Taiwan, all expenses paid, to develop a safety program starting at the elementary level. I turned them down.

365.2422

Then Gloria was promoted to CFO, which meant she would be working year-round at the home office in Seattle. It was a big change in our marriage. Before we met, I'd attended a doctoral candidate's defense of his dissertation, "Buckets of Love." In many relationships, he explained, each partner is looking for someone to fill their love bucket, and hopefully each person has what the other one lacks. The best combination, however, is two partners with full love buckets. Gloria and I were one of those lucky and hardworking couples. We were independent, secure people choosing to be interdependent in a relationship yet happy on our own. We both had gamma personalities; I lean a little to the alpha side and Gloria a little to the beta. We accepted each other unconditionally and were guided by our beliefs, passions, and priorities, and we both knew how to give love and receive love.

It was the first full year we were together. No time to just be us as individuals alone. No passionate reunions in the fall. No summer stories to swap. Our marriage was never in peril, but this change did warrant more than one "Let's have a glass of wine and talk" conversation. Once we adapted, our marriage was stronger than before.

Around this time, Gloria entered her midthirties and felt the clock ticking. "What if I regret not having children?" she asked. She'd entered my children's lives when they were nearly grown, and I made one big mistake early on. On the first Mother's Day after our marriage, she seemed a little blue. When I asked why, she said, "You didn't give me a Mother's Day card." I said the absolutely wrong thing: "You're not a mother." Boy, was that a mistake. She and the kids loved one another as much as anyone with or without shared blood.

As luck would have it, we had friends with a five-month-old daughter, Casey. They asked us if we would take care of her while they were in Japan on business. Waking up to comfort Casey after a nightmare, making sure she ate at least one green thing a day, getting her to and from day care on time—we had to pay fifty dollars once because we didn't pick her up on time—gave Gloria a taste of the reality of caring for little kids. She immediately turned off the clock.

A LIFE TOGETHER

How can I begin to describe nearly forty years of marriage?

Gloria's family of origin did not express love, and so I worked every day to let her know just how amazing she was, how loveable and kind and beautiful inside and out. My kids became her kids—they adored her. Vicki enlisted in the navy and served in the navy reserves, working in Seattle while waiting for admittance to dental technician school. She was stationed in San Diego as a dental tech, then used her GI Bill to attend Brigham Young University. She met her husband, Kevin Hansen, while working on her master's of library and information of science degree at the University of Washington. For their first date, Vicki told me and Gloria to get lost so she could use our kitchen to make dinner, which she accidentally set on fire. "Don't worry," we told her when we got home. "You'll probably marry him and laugh about it for the rest of your lives." She did and they do.

Scott got his start hacking into Stanford's early computer system, and, not surprisingly, he went on to work as a computer programmer. Susan graduated in 1978 and began working as an administrative assistant. She was married to the love of her life, Mike Talley, for five years before he died of stomach cancer.

The night my son Kevin turned eighteen, the union guys

took him to the International Alliance of Theatrical Stage Employees union meeting to be inducted into the union. He'd go on to work in all the professional theaters in Seattle, managing sets and sound systems for musicals and operas, ballets and symphonies, movies, concerts, and conventions. He was the prop manager at 5th Avenue Theater for many years, and he even went on a national tour with Debbie Reynolds for *The Unsinkable Molly Brown.*

Bonnie graduated from Rex College in Rexburg, Idaho, with a degree in audiology and speech pathology. She met and married Jack Feterrolf, an officer in the coast guard stationed in Seattle, in May 1977. She was pregnant with our first granddaughter when Gloria and I got married.

Over the years, Gloria spoiled her fourteen grandkids and nine great-grandkids silly. She saw the best in people, brought out the best in them, and, with her, it didn't take long for strangers to become friends. She loved sports, playing in a woman's tackle football league, and whenever anyone said a word against the Seahawks, she'd say, "Now, don't you talk about my boys like that!" Our life was simple and, in its way, perfect. Which doesn't necessarily make the best story—for story, you need conflict, and we managed to settle our rare differences with a glass of wine and a chat. It came down to the fact that she supported me, and I supported her. After our first Valentine's Day, not a day went by without us saying "I love you."

Gloria got sick in 2014. I knew it was serious when the surgery to address her stomach cancer went way beyond its scheduled duration. For the next three years, I did everything I could to make her comfortable. It was hard on me to be so useless, to watch her suffer and be able to do nothing about it. Of course, it was harder on her, but she rarely complained, and I never saw her cry. I wonder if she'd been trying to spare *me* pain—that was so like her.

We went on a two-week cruise a year into her illness, which had slowed us down but didn't stop us from enjoying life. (She could no longer drink wine, so she told me that we should try not to get upset with each other, because we couldn't "have a glass of wine and talk.") When school let out for the summer in 2016, we took our grandkids on a trip to Bryce Canyon National Park. Gloria had found out that they had not been to the park founded by their great-great-great-great-grandfather, and she was determined to remedy the situation. Though she was too tired to walk very far, she joined the rowdy group to ride horseback down into the canyon.

Two months before she died, an overgrown, weed-infested jungle that she had spent ten years shepherding into a gorgeous community trail in Shoreline was officially named Gloria's Path. The meeting hall was packed with friends, and several people got up to speak in her honor. My favorite was: "I would be honored to walk any path Gloria has walked."

Gloria stood to address the city council. Her only nutrition came through a feeding tube, and she was very weak. I stood and took her hand to walk with her up to the podium, then stepped back so she could deliver her speech: "I am very honored and humbled. Ever since I served on the original committee to make Shoreline a city, my heart has been in Shoreline. I've always felt that every citizen needs to contribute to where we live, and when this opportunity presented itself, it was meant for me to be a cheerleader with the neighbors and have them come and help."

When she was near the end, I asked her if she wanted some of her ashes to be spread on Gloria's Path. "No!" she said with as much energy as she could muster. "I don't want dogs pooping on me." She was funny, and warm and kind and generous, until her very last breath.

Gloria J. Kortus Bryce passed away on March 18, 2017. She

had been bedridden since late January, and we had spent our favorite holiday in bed, in each other's arms. I held her as close as I could without hurting her, trying to convey forty years' worth of love. I sure loved that gal.

On Valentine's Day of 2021, almost four years after Gloria's death and a year into the COVID-19 pandemic, I decided to work on my taxes. I had nothing better to do. During my search for a new ribbon for the calculator, I rifled through what I'd always thought of as her private drawer. There, at the back, was a Valentine's Day card from 2017. In it, she'd written, *You're still my best friend in the whole wide world. Being married to you has been marvelous.*

These days, when it's not too rainy, I walk Gloria's Path, thinking about my long and productive life, my parents and grandparents, my children and grandchildren and great-grandchildren. I think of Gloria, my beautiful wife, the love of my life.

EPILOGUE

Today, as I write this, I am eighty-eight years old. I am the great-great-grandson of Ebenezer and Mary Ann Park Bryce, early settlers of the area around Bryce Canyon. In 1882, they resettled in Arizona's Gila River Valley, across the Gila River from Pima, and named it Bryce.

I was born nearby on the San Carlos Indian Reservation in Geronimo, Arizona, which is now at the bottom of the San Carlos Reservoir behind Coolidge Dam. It was 1933, the worst year of the Great Depression for Arizona, and this set my bar for happiness and a good life very low. My father was a self-taught jack-of-all-*labor*-trades and followed the work, be it copper and silver mining, building a dam, logging maintenance, farming, auto repair, or building aircraft during World War II. I spent my formative years on my maternal grandparents' subsistence farm in a community of a dozen farms or so. Uncle Dewey's store/post office/gas station was the only place to buy anything, and the grade school also served as a church. We had no plumbing; water was brought in a large tank and transferred to a thousand-gallon cistern. My family was considered upper class because we had a three-holer out-house. When you start at this level, there is nowhere to go but up.

My grandparents had eleven children—two died in infancy—and I was honorary number twelve. They had a lot of hands-on experience raising kids, and they did it right. Grandpa attended only first and second grade, and Grandma's formal schooling ended after seventh, but they taught me everything I'd need to know in life: that love was the most important thing. I was Grandma's little helper, and I got loads of hugs, thank-yous, and kisses on my forehead. When I was older, I became Grandpa's little farmer. He gave me chores, which he called "jobs," to earn my room and board, such as collecting the eggs, feeding the chickens and rabbits, and bringing in kindling for Grandma's woodstove. I was free to roam, as long as I stayed off the paved highway and was back before supper. If I wanted candy, I could take some eggs down to Dewey's store and trade them. When I asked how or why something worked, Grandpa took the time to teach me. When I did something wrong, as little boys occasionally do, no one called me a bad boy or told me I was stupid. Instead, they helped me understand why it was wrong.

This was my world, my measuring stick. I was happy and made to feel important. I was loved and trusted, and I learned how to love and maintain trust in return. I understood that I was a part of the whole, that I was responsible for my actions and had to pull my weight and it was my duty to give more than take. I developed a strong self-confidence, which I realized, later in life, means recognizing your limits as well. My grandparents and my father awakened my scientific mind. Of course, I didn't understand all that at that age. In truth, writing my first book, *Me and the Cottonwood Tree: An Untethered Boyhood*, made me understand the impact my grandparents had on me.

Life wasn't perfect, of course. I've experienced as much grief as anyone. At the time of this writing, I am the oldest person on my mom's side and the second oldest living Bryce— surpassed only by my dad's youngest brother, Ed—meaning I've lost all those people who took such good care of me. I've seen injustice and racism and a whole lot of change and life's general unfairness. I've had to get comfortable with mysteries that never get solved, questions that never get answered.

Teaching science has been an absolute joy, and getting to see how my students take what they learned in my classrooms and use it to succeed in life—that's the greatest reward. My five children are the highlight of my life, as are my fourteen grandkids, and thirteen great-grandkids and counting. I can only hope that I passed down a smidgen of the wisdom my grandparents shared with me. I've learned from my kids and grandkids and great-grandkids, again, that love has no limits. Gloria, my wife of forty years, taught me the same lesson. I am forever grateful that we found each other. As a scientific realist, I believe it was a series of unintended incidents that brought us together. Gloria thought it was fate. Whatever it was, we were soul mates for all those decades, changing and falling in love again and again.

To quote Mae West: "You only live once, but if you do it right, once is enough." My life has been extraordinary and or- dinary, as all lives are. I worked hard and enjoyed the beauty the world has to offer. Mae West was right, once is enough.

ACKNOWLEDGMENTS

Another sincere thank you to Anna Katz. We had as good a time working on the second book as we did the first, and now she knows all my secrets. I am grateful for her thoughtfulness, her deep listening, and her ability to turn almost ninety years' worth of experience into a story.

ABOUT THE AUTHOR

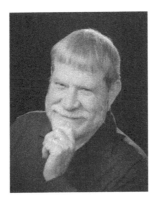

Photo © Lifetouch

Herb Bryce was born in rural Arizona in 1933 and moved extensively throughout his childhood and teenage years. After serving four years in the Navy during the Korean War, he entered Arizona State University, where he received his undergraduate and graduate degrees. He pursued a career in the sciences, notably as division chair of Physical Sciences at Citrus College and as the dean of Science and Mathematics at Seattle Central College. Herb was highly active in the American Chemical Society and served on the Shoreline School Board and on the Shoreline Parks, Recreation, and Cultural Services board for many years. He has a passion for the arts and is a cofounder and board member of ShoreLake Arts.

In his spare time, Herb loves to travel to gain an understanding of cultures around the world. Herb currently lives in Shoreline, Washington, where he is an active member of his local community. His philosophy is that service is the rent we pay for living. *Beyond the Cottonwood Trees* is Herb's second memoir. Please visit the author at www.HerbBryce.com.